Dietitian's Guide
to
Assessment
and
Documentation

Jacqueline C. Morris, RD, MPH, CDN

Executive Director, Annex Nutrition Services
Elmsford, New York

JONES AND BARTLETT PUBLISHERS
Sudbury, Massachusetts
BOSTON   TORONTO   LONDON   SINGAPORE

Jones and Bartlett Publishers
40 Tall Pine Drive
Sudbury, MA 01776
978-443-5000
info@jbpub.com
www.jbpub.com

Jones and Bartlett Publishers
Canada
6339 Ormindale Way
Mississauga, Ontario L5V 1J2
Canada

Jones and Bartlett Publishers
International
Barb House, Barb Mews
London W6 7PA
United Kingdom

Jones and Bartlett's books and products are available through most bookstores and online booksellers. To contact Jones and Bartlett Publishers directly, call 800-832-0034, fax 978-443-8000, or visit our website, www.jbpub.com.

Substantial discounts on bulk quantities of Jones and Bartlett's publications are available to corporations, professional associations, and other qualified organizations. For details and specific discount information, contact the special sales department at Jones and Bartlett via the above contact information or send an email to specialsales@jbpub.com.

The author, editor, and publisher have made every effort to provide accurate information. However, they are not responsible for errors, omissions, or for any outcomes related to the use of the contents of this book and take no responsibility for the use of the products and procedures described. Treatments and side effects described in this book may not be applicable to all people; likewise, some people may require a dose or experience a side effect that is not described herein. Drugs and medical devices are discussed that may have limited availability controlled by the Food and Drug Administration (FDA) for use only in a research study or clinical trial. Research, clinical practice, and government regulations often change the accepted standard in this field. When consideration is being given to use of any drug in the clinical setting, the health care provider or reader is responsible for determining FDA status of the drug, reading the package insert, and reviewing prescribing information for the most up-to-date recommendations on dose, precautions, and contraindications, and determining the appropriate usage for the product. This is especially important in the case of drugs that are new or seldom used.

Production Credits

Publisher: David Cella
Acquisitions Editor: Katey Birtcher
Associate Editor: Maro Gartside
Editorial Assistant: Teresa Reilly
Senior Production Editor: Renée Sekerak
Production Assistant: Jill Morton
Marketing Manager: Grace Richards
Manufacturing and Inventory Control Supervisor: Amy Bacus

Composition: Abella Publishing Services
Cover and Title Page Design: Scott Moden
Cover Image: © Designus/ShutterStock, Inc.
Printing and Binding: Malloy Incorporated
Cover Printing: Malloy Incorporated

Library of Congress Cataloging-in-Publication Data
Morris, Jacqueline C.
  Dietitian's guide to assessment and documentation / by Jacqueline C. Morris.
    p. ; cm.
  Includes bibliographical references and index.
  ISBN-13: 978-0-7637-7851-4
  ISBN-10: 0-7637-7851-6
  1. Nutrition--Evaluation. 2. Medical history taking. I. Title.
  [DNLM: 1. Nutrition Assessment. 2. Diet Therapy--methods. 3. Medical History Taking. 4. Nutritional Physiological Phenomena--physiology. 5. Patient Education as Topic. QU 146.1 M872d 2011]
  RC621.M67 2011
  613.2072--dc22
                              2009044805
6048
Printed in the United States of America
14 13 12 11 10   10 9 8 7 6 5 4 3 2 1

Contents

Foreword vii

Preface ix

Introduction xi

Acknowledgments xiii

About the Author xv

Reviewers xvii

PART 1   Identifying the Problem: Collecting and
             Analyzing the Evidence 1

Chapter 1   Chart Review 3
             Medical Diagnosis 4
             Surgical Review and History 5
             Weight History 12
             Skin Integrity 15
             Gastrointestinal Review 17
             Cardiovascular Review 28
             Psychiatric Review 33
             Infectious Diseases 34
             Musculoskeletal Review 40
             Psychosocial Review .41
             Pulmonary Review 41
             Biochemical Data Review 43
             Review of Medications 43

Chapter 2	**The Interview** **59**
	Obtaining Diet History 60
	Obtaining Weight History. .61
	24-Hour Recall 62
	Food Frequency Questionnaire 62
	The Relationship Between
	Race/Ethnicity and Diseases 63
	Understanding Culture and Dietary Practices 64
	Religion and Food Practices. 66
	The Use of Herbal Supplements. 69
	Food Allergy and Intolerance 74

Chapter 3	**Objective Tools to Collect Information**
	for Assessment **81**
	Direct Observation Study. .81
	Calorie Count Study 82
	Body Mass Index. 85
	Waist Circumference and Waist-to-Hip Ratio 86
	Body Fat Percentage. 86
	Indirect Calorimetry. 88
	Nitrogen Balance 89
	Bone Mineral Density Test 90

Chapter 4	**Assessment During Pregnancy and Lactation. . . . 93**
	Dietary Assessment of the Pregnant Woman 93
	Nutritional Needs of the Pregnant Woman 96
	Weight Gain During Pregnancy. 98
	Risk Factors for Fetal Growth Retardation. 99
	Complications in Pregnancy and
	Dietary Intervention. 100
	Lactation 103

Chapter 5	**Pediatric Assessment. 107**
	Assessing the Newborn. 107
	Nutritional Care of the Low-Birthweight Infant. . .108
	Assessing the Full-Term Infant. 112
	Failure to Thrive. 112
	Mental Retardation and
	Developmental Disability. 116

Inborn Errors of Amino Acid Metabolism. 117
Eating Disorders in Children and Adolescents . . .119
Pediatric Obesity. 123

PART II   Solving the Problem:
               Creating a Plan of Care 129

Chapter 6   Determining Nutrient Requirements
               and Writing the Care Plan 131
               Determining Fluid Needs. 132
               Creating a Plan of Care 134

Chapter 7   Patient Teaching. 145
               Writing Learning Objectives 149
               Evaluating Patient Teaching. 149

Chapter 8   Diet Teaching for Specific Medical Conditions . . .153

PART III   Documentation 169

Chapter 9   The Legal Aspects of Documentation 171
               Why Document? 171
               The Purpose of Documentation. 171
               The Medical Record as a Legal Document. 172
               Common Documentation Issues
                  in Malpractice Lawsuits 172
               General Information Regarding Documentation . . .174
               Mechanics of Good Documentation 176
               Documentation Using the Nutrition Care Process. .178

               Appendix 181
               Approved Abbreviation List for Some
                  Common Diagnoses and Terms. 181

               Index 193

Foreword

This book does not pretend to encompass all aspects of general nutrition. Nevertheless, the author, driven to face with confidence the daily challenges of clinical nutrition, has embarked on arduous work that results in a very concise, yet comprehensive resource aimed at the generalist, dietitian or nutritionist, gastroenterologist, and student.

The objective is to bring forward current and emerging evidence regarding nutrition assessment and documentation. For example, obesity has attained epidemic proportions worldwide. In the United States, more than 30% of adults and 15% of children are obese and consequently are at risk for more than 36 different medical conditions. Premature deaths from obesity are approximately 300,000 annually; consumer expenditures for weight loss products are $45 billion; healthcare expenses for obesity are more than $100 billion per year. Malnutrition, on the other hand, although less prevalent than obesity, is a serious clinical issue in patients with HIV infection and other chronic clinical conditions such as liver cirrhosis.

These facts prompted a revolution in methods of nutritional assessment of the individual, and dietary and nutritional interactions with the disease aimed at changing the natural history and improving the quality of life. This process continues to evolve.

Jacqueline Morris has spent countless hours compiling the evidence to provide an efficient and meaningful learning experience. The book is organized into nine chapters, and elegantly provides information on core methods of nutritional assessment, diagnosis, approaches to management of weight gain and malnutrition, nutritional support, efficient documentation, and reasonable prevention. A full table of contents and references are provided for the convenience of the reader. I am certain readers will enjoy this book and find it extremely useful in designing nutrition assessments and documenting the nutrition health of individual patients.

Prospere Remy, MD
Chief, Gastroenterology and Liver Disease
Bronx Lebanon Hospital Center
Bronx, New York

Preface

Delivering nutrition care to your patient is a four-step process as outlined by the American Dietetic Association's Nutrition Care Process:

1. Nutrition assessment
2. Nutrition diagnosis
3. Nutrition intervention
4. Nutrition monitoring and evaluation

Before you identify the problem or potential nutrition risk(s), it is important that you first review the medical chart, which gives information about the patient: diagnosis, social history, medical history, medication, laboratory data and assessment, and evaluations performed by other medical/clinical personnel. Reading the notes of other clinicians who have documented information about the patient provides necessary context for effective management of the condition(s) being assessed. Dietitians in private practice obtain this information from the referring physician and the patient or family.

The next step is to interview the patient to obtain diet history and other pertinent data to determine a solution to the existing problem or means by which to reduce the risk of a potential problem. With a chart review and patient interview, you can identify the nutrition problem and its etiology and provide nutrition intervention to address that problem.

To provide the appropriate intervention to meet the nutritional needs of the patient, you must have a clear understanding of the medical diagnosis and its nutritional implications. Once intervention is initiated, you must carefully monitor the patient to ensure that goals are met and the desired outcome is achieved.

Documenting findings, interventions, and outcomes in the medical record is critical to the nutrition care process—notes should paint a clear picture without ambiguity. Details of proper documentation and steps in the delivery of nutrition care to the patient are covered throughout this book.

I have had the opportunity to present this topic to dietitians on multiple occasions and was quite impressed with the outcome of the evaluations. I believe it is helpful to have this information available to everyone in the field of dietetics and nutrition, especially new dietitians. It can also sharpen the skills of those already in practice. The materials in this book have been carefully reviewed by physicians and peers, and I hope you will find it a useful and helpful resource.

Introduction

The dietitian plays a critical role in the delivery of care to the patient. As an integral part of the healthcare team, you are responsible for helping to maintain good health and quality of life for the patients and clients you serve so well. You are more than just the "food person" that many make you out to be. You consult with physicians and other healthcare professionals to ensure the best possible outcome for their patients. However, as you execute your duties and responsibilities as a dietitian, it is extremely important that you keep abreast of the ever-changing science of medicine and nutrition because some information that you learned in school is no longer applicable today. You must have a working knowledge of the disease state that is being assessed.

To provide patients and clients with optimal care, dietitians must go below the surface and think like investigators, which is what they really are. The dietitian's work can be described as that of a "nutritional status investigator." While investigating the nutritional status of your patients/clients and implementing care, you must be careful to document with the law in mind because you never know when you will be called to defend what you wrote. Good documentation can keep you out of court as well as defend you in an investigation or a malpractice lawsuit.

The purpose of this book is to give details of the components of nutrition care assessment, referred to by the American Dietetic Association as the Nutrition Care Process, and to provide information on the legal aspects of documentation. It is intended to be used in collaboration with other texts that outline the nutrition care process as indicated by the American Dietetic Association. You are probably quite familiar with the phrase "if it is not documented, it was not done." This book will help you avoid the pitfalls of improper documentation.

This book also provides an overview of common diseases and their effect on nutritional status, as well as a clear understanding of biochemical data and categories of medications as they relate to health and diseases. Included in this book you can find important information on patient teaching for specific medical conditions and acceptable abbreviations used in health care.

Acknowledgments

I would like to personally thank my friends, colleagues, and family whose support and encouragement made the publication of this book possible.

I would like to thank Sarah Barnes, my fellow dietitian, who first recommended me to speak on the topic of nutrition assessment and documentation to a group of more than 200 dietitians at the League 1199 Training and Upgrading Fund in 2005. This opportunity gave me the confidence to pursue writing this book, which is to be made available to new dietitians and to sharpen the skills of those with years of practice in dietetics and nutrition.

Special thanks to those who reviewed and edited the contents of this book. I am especially grateful to Prospere Remy, MD, chief of Gastroenterology and Liver Disease, Bronx Lebanon Hospital Center; Karen Formato, RD, director of Clinical Nutrition, Bronx Lebanon Hospital Center; MaryAlice Laub, RD, CNSD; Richard Tennant, RN; Maurice Harbon, PharmD; Geoffrey Lord, PharmD; and Arlene Spark, EdD, RD, FADA, FACN, coordinator of Nutrition at Hunter College.

I would like to acknowledge two of my good friends, Vixton Dixton and Samuel King, who always believed in me and provided support in the establishment of Annex Nutrition Services.

Thanks to my mom, Dorothy Brady, for her prayerful support; my dad and siblings, for being there for me. Thanks to my step-son, Matthew, for helping with the typing.

I especially want to thank Claudette Beckford, LD, and Sarah Addoyobo, RD, CDN, MS, from Richmond Strategy, Inc. (formerly Richmond Children Center) for giving me my first opportunity to practice dietetics in New York. Thanks also to my preceptors at Danbury Hospital where I completed my dietetic internship.

Last, I would like to thank my patients, former employers, and current clients, who gave me the opportunity to grow and expand my expertise. I learned a lot from both my patients and colleagues.

About the Author

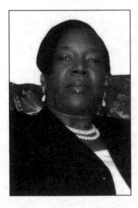

Jacqueline C. Morris, RD, MPH, CDN, hails from the beautiful island of Jamaica, where she started her career in dietetics and nutrition. She graduated from the University of Technology in 1986 with an associate degree in Food, Nutrition, and Dietetics. She worked as an assistant dietitian at Falmouth Hospital and taught food and nutrition to high school students.

In 1993, she migrated to the United States, where she pursued her bachelor's degree in nutrition at Lehman College and later earned a Master of Public Health degree from New York University.

She was the editor of the *Beth Israel Cancer Center Newsletter*, to which she also contributed several nutrition articles, including "'Phyte' Back with Phytochemicals." She worked as a clinical nutrition manager at the Bronx Lebanon Special Care Center for a number of years and developed educational materials for both staff and patients.

In 2003, Ms. Morris started her own consulting firm, Annex Nutrition Services, in Elmsford, New York. Annex Nutrition Services offers continuing education credits to dietitians, nurses, dietetic technicians, and students, as well as private counseling both at home and in the office setting. Ms. Morris works in collaboration with other companies to provide wellness programs at the corporate level and is a service provider for various healthcare agencies.

Reviewers

Jo Carol Chezem, PhD, RD
Associate Professor of Nutrition
Ball State University
Muncie, IN

B. J. Friedman, PhD, RD, LD
Professor, Director, Texas State Dietetic Internship
Texas State University
San Marcos, TX

Kathleen M. Laquale, PhD, ATC, LAT, LDN
Professor
Bridgewater State College
Bridgewater, MA

Tania Rivera, MS, RD, LD/N
Assistant Clinical Professor
Florida International University
Miami, FL

Identifying the Problem

Collecting and Analyzing the Evidence

Chart Review

A thorough nutrition assessment begins with a review of the patient's medical chart. The medical chart provides information on the patient's medical history, diagnosis or diagnoses, physical assessment, treatment, laboratory data, medications, social history, and response to treatment. This chapter reviews the various systems, their nutritional implications, and intervention.

The Nutrition Care Process according to the American Dietetic Association involves four steps:

1. *Nutrition assessment*: The nutrition assessment is a systematic approach used to collect, record, and interpret relevant data from patients, clients, family members, caregivers, and other individuals and groups. It takes into consideration anthropometric data, diet/ medical history, biochemical data, and social history.
2. *Nutrition diagnosis*: The nutrition diagnosis is the diagnosis of nutrition-related problems based on signs and symptoms from the assessment data.

3. *Nutrition intervention:* The nutrition intervention is a plan designed to address the nutrition diagnosis for which goals are developed with the patient/client and reviewed for modification as needed.
4. *Nutrition monitoring and evaluation:* This step identifies the progress made on the plan of care and measures outcomes.

In reviewing the patient's medical record, it is important you have a clear understanding of the medical diagnosis(es) and its impact on nutritional status, food–drug interaction, and laboratory values. These topics are covered in detail in this chapter.

MEDICAL DIAGNOSIS

Medical diagnosis varies from one patient to another, and some patients present with multiple diagnoses. In assessing the patient's nutritional status, you often can find that for some patients one diagnosis takes precedence over another. The diagnosis is pivotal to your assessment. For example, you review the chart of a patient who has a diagnosis of hypertension, but also has poor oral intake. As a dietitian, your primary focus is to ensure adequate caloric intake, and in this case, that might mean offering a regular diet instead of a sodium-restricted diet so as to encourage good oral intake.

Let's say JB is admitted to your facility with a history of hepatic encephalopathy and has severe depletion of albumin with wasting syndrome. Instead of reducing protein intake because of the hepatic encephalopathy, your focus now shifts to the low albumin and wasting syndrome. The goal, therefore, is to provide adequate protein and calories to improve nutritional status. Lactulose/neomycin is usually administered to decrease the ammonia level and subsequently improve hepatic encephalopathy.

I remember some years ago during my internship, I encountered a patient who was diagnosed with cancer, but who also had diabetes. I went into his room because I had received a nutrition consult for diabetes management. I put all my instruction sheets together and was ready to show off my counseling skills.

His wife was with him as I entered the room. I introduced myself and began sharing my expertise in diabetes management when his wife said, "We are not worried about his diabetes; that is the least of our concerns.

My husband has cancer." I realized then that the diagnosis that concerned her most was cancer, and therefore the couple was not prepared to receive counseling on managing diabetes. It is important to listen to your patient to determine learning readiness.

You can never be familiar with all the diagnoses that exist, but when in doubt, "check it out." Make use of the physicians on your team and get a better understanding of the diagnoses because in almost all cases, nutrition plays a vital role in the recovery process. Whatever the diagnosis, the aim is to provide adequate nutrition to reduce the risk of malnutrition because malnutrition slows recovery time for patients. Sometimes it becomes necessary to focus on the diagnosis with the greatest impact on the patient's medical and nutritional health.

SURGICAL REVIEW AND HISTORY

Some, if not all, surgical procedures have a direct impact on patients' nutritional status and outcome. Surgery is almost always accompanied by weight loss resulting from fasting before the procedure and decreased oral intake immediately following the procedure. It is not unusual for a patient's hemoglobin, hematocrit, and albumin levels to fall significantly following surgery. This section highlights some common surgical procedures and their nutritional implications.

Gastric Bypass Surgery

In an effort to manage weight, many obese individuals turn to surgical procedures. In recent years, the number of gastric bypass surgeries being performed yearly has increased. According to the Centers for Disease Control and Prevention (CDC), more than 60% of Americans are overweight, and about 3 in 10 are obese. Gastric bypass involves reducing the size of the stomach by applying rows of stainless steel staples across the top of the stomach so that only a small opening into the distal stomach is left open. This is then connected to the small intestine by means of an intestinal loop (Mahan & Escott-Stump, 2008).

Nutritional Implications and Intervention

Gastric bypass surgery patients take in less food and absorb less of what they ingest, putting them at risk for developing nutritional deficiencies.

Bloating, nausea, and vomiting are common in these patients. The goal of nutrition therapy is to maximize nutritional intake in small quantities and prevent "dumping syndrome," which occurs when food passes too quickly from the stomach to the small intestine. Symptoms of dumping syndrome may include feelings of nausea, feelings of fullness, stomach cramping, diarrhea, weakness, sweating, and a fast heart rate.

Another complication of gastric bypass surgery is the formation of gallstones, which frequently leads to the need for gallbladder surgery. Most surgeons remove the gallbladder during the gastric bypass surgery to prevent this from happening. Patients should be monitored for potential anemia and deficiencies of potassium, magnesium, folate, and vitamin B_{12}. Vitamin and mineral supplements are necessary for life following surgery.

Short Bowel Syndrome

Short bowel syndrome is often the result of extensive intestinal resection and is characterized by diarrhea, malabsorption, and malnutrition related to a shortened intestinal remnant. "Patients who are at the greatest nutritional and dehydration risk generally have < 115 cm of residual small intestine in the absence of colon in continuity or < 60 cm of residual small intestine with colon in continuity" (Buchman, 2004).

Hydration and nutritional status are difficult to maintain without nutrition support when more than 75% of the small intestine has been resected. To assess the nutritional status of patients with short bowel syndrome effectively, you need to know the extent of the resection, whether the ileocecal valve was removed, which segment of the small bowel remains, and the adaptation potential of the remaining gut. "An intact colon may absorb up to 1200 cal/day" (Buchman, 2004).

Nutritional Implications and Intervention

With extensive ileal resections, the proximal gut does not gain the capacity to absorb bile salts or vitamin B_{12}, and the ileal "brake" on upper gut transit is lost. Removal of the ileocecal valve may lead to bacterial overgrowth. As a consequence of these abnormalities, progressive dehydration, hypovolemia, electrolyte imbalances, and malabsorption of fat, fat-soluble vitamins (A, D, E, and K), vitamin B_{12} and divalent cations (calcium, magnesium, zinc, and copper) may develop (Bernard, 1993).

Anemia resulting from vitamin B_{12} deficiency in patients with short bowel syndrome (SBS) is believed to be linked to *Lactobacillus* overgrowth; lactobacilli require vitamin B_{12}, for growth (Hojo Bando, Itoh, Taketomo, & Ishii, 2008).

One of the major complications of short bowel syndrome is chronic diarrhea resulting from malabsorption. After massive small bowel resection, increased gastrointestinal losses can often cause dehydration, hyponatremia, hypokalemia, hypomagnesemia, hypocalcemia, and metabolic acidosis. Most patients require total parenteral nutrition (TPN) for 7 to 10 days following the resection. Energy requirements are generally 25–35 cal/kg/day, and protein requirements are 1.0–1.5g/kg/day.

Patients may also experience steatorrhea, and MCT oil is usually recommended to enhance absorption of nutrients. MCT oil, however, lacks linoleic acid, an essential fatty acid. Plant oils, for example, safflower and sunflower, are good sources of linoleic acid. Reducing fat intake helps to decrease steatorrhea.

Fluid requirements are modified to prevent dehydration. You must, however, monitor fluid status daily for clinical signs of fluid overload or dehydration. Oral rehydration solutions (ORSs) are recommended to reduce sodium loss.

The goal of nutrition therapy for the patient with short bowel syndrome is to ensure adequate fluid and electrolyte replacement, stabilize diarrhea, prevent loss of or replace water-soluble and fat-soluble vitamins, and prevent vitamin B_{12} deficiency. Vitamin K deficiency may occur in patients who do not have a colon because colonic bacteria synthesize 60% of daily vitamin K requirements.

Patients with short bowel syndrome who do not receive TPN are generally in negative calcium balance, and you should prescribe a supplement (800–1500 mg/day) (Buchman, 2004).

If the colon is intact, the patient is at increased risk of developing calcium oxalate renal stones. Patients presenting with calcium oxalate kidney stones should restrict dietary oxalate. Foods high in oxalate include tea, cola drinks, chocolate, nuts, green leafy vegetables, celery, strawberries, blueberries, and tangerines. Frequent meals consisting of complex carbohydrate and soluble fiber are strongly encouraged in the patient with an intact colon.

Missing Body Parts

From time to time, a patient will present to your facility with missing body parts, whether it be an arm, a leg, or even a breast. Because breast size varies from one woman to another and body weight differs among patients, it is important to ascertain the patient's body weight prior to mastectomy and after mastectomy when the patient resumes a normal eating pattern because weight loss immediately after surgery might be a combination of breast tissue loss as well as blood and fluid loss.

Amputations

You can calculate the patient's approximate body weight loss following an amputation by using this list as a guide:

Hand represents	0.7% loss	Foot represents	1.5% loss
Forearm with hand represents	2.3% loss	Lower leg and foot represents	6.0% loss
Entire arm represents	5.0% loss	Entire leg represents	16.0% loss

Nutritional Implications and Intervention

Missing body parts affect the estimated caloric and protein needs of the patient. To determine the ideal body weight (IBW) of the patient with a missing body part, first establish the IBW prior to amputation, and then subtract the percentage of the missing body part as well as the weight of any prostheses.

Coronary Artery Bypass Grafting Surgery

When a coronary artery becomes narrowed or clogged, the section of the heart that it supplies suffers. Coronary artery bypass grafting surgery (CABG) is a way to treat the blocked artery by creating new passages for blood to flow to the heart muscles. It works by taking arteries or veins from other parts of the body, called grafts, and using them to reroute blood around the clogged artery. Coronary artery bypass grafting surgery, however, does not cure atherosclerosis because the new grafts are susceptible to atherogenesis, the formation of plaques in the inner lining of the arteries (Mahan & Escott-Stump, 2008).

This surgical procedure is increasingly performed in older adults who are vulnerable to undernutrition. Among the risk factors associated with adverse outcomes are low serum albumin and body mass index (BMI). Rich et al. retrospectively analyzed the effect of hypoalbuminemia (serum albumin level < 3.5 g/dL) on postoperative complications in 92 patients (> 75 years of age) undergoing cardiac surgery over a 2-year period. Fourteen percent were hypoalbuminemic, and hypoalbuminemia was the most significant predictor of postoperative renal dysfunction and a contributor to postoperative length of stay. Patients classified as having hypoalbuminemia, hypoalbuminemia and liver insufficiency, or hypoalbuminemia and congestive heart failure had an increased likelihood of postoperative organ dysfunction, gastrointestinal bleeding, nosocomial infections, extended length of intensive care unit stay, prolonged duration of mechanical ventilation, and hospital death.

"In another series of 886 Swedish cardiac surgery patients (63% were ≥ 65 years of age), a low preoperative serum albumin level was also associated with an increased rate of postoperative infection, and a low preoperative BMI increased the risk for death. Engleman et al. also demonstrated that low preoperative serum albumin level (< 2.5 g/dL) and low BMI (< 20 kg/m²) independently predicted mortality after cardiac surgery" (DiMaria-Ghalili, 2008).

> DiMaria-Ghalili systematically examined the relationship between nutrition markers (BMI, serum albumin, and transferrin levels) before surgery and again at 4–5 days post-surgery and 4–6 weeks post-discharge, as well as biomedical and general health outcomes, in 91 elderly patients undergoing elective CABG surgery. Although older patients undergoing elective CABG had a normal preoperative nutrition status, weight loss during the later phases of the surgical stress response was problematic. Older patients undergoing elective CABG lost an average of 5.2% ± 4.3% of their weight from pre-surgery to 6 weeks post-discharge. The more weight lost during this period, the lower their level of self-reported physical health and the greater their chances of being readmitted to the hospital. Thus, older CABG patients who lose weight in the postoperative period may increase their vulnerability to adverse health outcomes, including hospital readmission." (DiMaria-Ghalili, 2008, Oct–Nov; *23* (5), 498)

Nutritional Implications and Intervention

To reduce the risk of mortality following cardiac surgery it is important that you conduct a thorough nutrition evaluation on the patient. Decreased dietary intake can lead to weight loss and subsequent malnutrition.

Depression is associated with decreased oral intake, decreased appetite, and weight loss. Weight loss especially in older adults correlates with increased mortality. Postoperative weight loss is also common in the CABG patient.

Like other postsurgical procedures, the postoperative CABG patient is put on a liquid diet that is low in fat and cholesterol until the individual is able to tolerate regular consistency. Patients are advised to follow a low-fat, low-cholesterol diet after discharge; however, because of the metabolic demands of CABG surgery, some surgeons advise patients not to make dietary changes until their appetite has returned to normal to ensure that adequate calories and proteins are consumed to promote recovery. This recommendation is appropriate because CABG patients frequently report decreased appetite and a change in the taste of food in the early weeks after discharge (DiMaria-Ghalili, 2008).

Pancreatectomy

The pancreas is the central organ for digestion and for control of glucose homeostasis. Whenever a patient experiences complications of chronic or acute pancreatitis or pancreatic malignancies, pancreatic surgery may be necessary. According to the National Cancer Institute, one of the following types of surgery may be used to remove tumors in the patient with pancreatic cancer:

- *Whipple procedure:* The head of the pancreas, the gallbladder, part of the stomach, part of the small intestine, and the bile duct are removed. Enough of the pancreas is left to produce digestive juices and insulin.
- *Total pancreatectomy:* The whole pancreas, part of the stomach, part of the small intestine, the common bile duct, the gallbladder, the spleen, and nearby lymph nodes are removed.
- *Distal pancreatectomy:* The body and the tail of the pancreas and usually the spleen are removed.

Nutritional Implications and Intervention

Most patients develop diabetes mellitus following pancreatectomy, requiring them to have insulin substitution. Hypoglycemia is the most difficult clinical problem to handle following pancreatectomy, and therefore carbohydrate intake must be adequate while monitoring blood glucose.

Alterations in glucagon regulation is considered a potential side effect of partial pancreatectomies (Schrader et al., 2009). Glucagon injection is administered when blood sugar drops significantly low.

Improvements in postoperative management include auto-islet cell transplantation, advances in insulin formulations, and the use of glucagon rescue therapy, which allow much tighter control of blood glucose than previously possible. This markedly lessens the risk of life-threatening hypoglycemia and decreases the risk of long-term complications, resulting in improved quality of life for these patients (Heidt, Burant, & Simeone, 2007).

The main clinical manifestations of exocrine pancreatic insufficiency are fat malabsorption, which is called steatorrhea and which consists of fecal excretion of more than 6 g per day of fat; weight loss; abdominal pain; and abdominal swelling sensation (Bini, 2007). There is also malabsorption of carbohydrates and protein, but fat malabsorption is more severe.

The presence of weight loss requires an increased energy intake. Dietary protein and carbohydrates should be high. Medium chain triglycerides (MCTs) are recommended for patients with steatorrhea because these fatty acids are hydrolyzed more rapidly.

The extent of malabsorption depends on the original disease process and the type and extent of surgical resection. Pancreatectomy interferes with the production of pancreatic enzymes necessary to digest nutrients, so to reduce the risk of malnutrition, pancreatic enzyme supplements (extracts) are given. The medical therapy target is to correct fat, protein, and carbohydrate malabsorption with pancreatic extracts, and secondary diabetes mellitus with insulin. Pancreatic extracts must be given with meals for good effect.

Ileostomy/Colostomy

An ostomy may be required when part of the urinary tract or bowel does not work and an alternate route must be created for the flow of waste. In the procedure, an opening called a stoma is surgically created between the body surface and the intestinal tract, allowing defecation from the intact portion of the intestine.

When the entire colon, rectum, and anus have to be removed following severe colitis, Crohn's disease, colon cancer, or intestinal trauma, an **ileostomy** or opening into the ileum is performed. If only the rectum and anus are removed, a **colostomy** can provide entrance to the colon.

The consistency of the stool from an ileostomy is liquid, whereas that from a colostomy ranges from mushy to fairy well formed. Odor is a major concern for the patient with an ileostomy or colostomy.

Nutritional Implications and Intervention

Foods that tend to cause odor from a colostomy are corn, dried beans, onions, cabbage, highly spiced foods, and fish. Fibrous vegetables should be avoided, and patients must chew foods well to prevent food getting caught at the point where the ileum narrows as it enters the abdominal wall, causing a food blockage.

Symptoms of blockage include the following:

- Objectionable odor
- Change in discharge from a semisolid to a thin liquid
- Increase in volume of output
- Cramping
- Distended abdomen
- Vomiting
- No ileostomy output, which usually occurs when there is complete blockage

Because of excessive losses of salt and water in patients with ileostomy, it is important that the diet be adequate in sodium and water. Electrolytes should be monitored closely. Gas-forming foods such as Brussels sprouts, peas, spinach, corn, cabbage, broccoli, string beans, dried beans, beer, cucumbers, carbonated beverages, and mushrooms should be limited.

If diarrhea occurs, the patient should follow a low-residue diet. Strained banana, applesauce, boiled rice, and tapioca are some foods that may help alleviate diarrhea.

WEIGHT HISTORY

The patient's weight is pivotal to the nutrition assessment. When a patient is first admitted to the hospital or nursing home, his or her ideal body weight is not the main concern because that patient might be overweight but still malnourished because of poor oral intake prior to admission. It is, therefore, important to ascertain the patient's usual body weight and compare that weight to the current weight to determine severity of weight loss, if any. Patients should be weighed on admission. If you are unable to obtain weight from the patient's chart, utilize family members to obtain an estimated weight until the accurate weight measurement is available. Should you decide to use an estimated weight based on visual assessment, or as reported by the patient or family members, you should document the term *estimated weight* or *reported weight* in the nutrition assessment. Make an effort to obtain the patient's correct weight as soon as possible after admission. Patients can be malnourished, yet present with normal weight because of fluid overload. Therefore, use the patient's ideal body weight to determine caloric and protein needs.

Height is important in determining ideal body weight. Ideally, the patient should be measured to obtain an accurate height; if you are unable to do so, using the height reported by the patient is acceptable. You can also obtain height information from the patient's driver's license. If you must estimate height then document it as *estimated height.*

Determining Ideal Body Weight

You can determine the ideal body weight by following these guides:

Male: Allow 106 pounds for the first 5 ft and 6 pounds for each additional inch.

Female: Allow 100 pounds for the first 5 ft and 5 pounds for each additional inch. If the patient is less than 5 ft, subtract 5 pounds for each inch shorter than 5 ft.

Always create a weight range, which is usually 10% below and 10% above ideal body weight. For example, a woman who is 5ft 5 in. tall would have a weight range of 113–138 pounds.

Determining Adjusted Body Weight

Adjusted body weight is used for patients whose current weight is greater than or equal to 125% of their ideal body weight. Today body mass index (BMI) is most commonly used to determine overweight and obesity status.

Formula:

$$(\text{Actual weight} - \text{Ideal body weight}) \times 25\% + \text{Ideal weight} = \text{Adjusted body weight}$$

Example: For a male 5 ft 8 in. tall who weighs 250 pounds, the calculation for adjusted body weight is as follows:

$$\text{Actual weight (250 pounds)} - \text{Ideal body weight (154 pounds)}$$
$$= 96 \text{ pounds}$$
$$96 \times .25 = 24 \text{ pounds}$$
$$24 + 154 = 178 \text{ pounds}$$
$$\text{Adjusted body weight} = 178 \text{ pounds}$$

Determining Weight Change

Here are the formulas for calculating weight changes:

- % Ideal body weight = Current weight ÷ Ideal body weight × 100
- % Usual body weight = Current weight ÷ usual body weight × 100
- % of Weight change = (Usual body weight − Current weight ÷ Usual body weight × 100)

UBW refers to previous weight at a specific point in time, for example, 1 month ago, or 6 months ago. **Table 1–1** shows guidelines on how to interpret weight changes.

Nutritional Implications and Intervention

Based on weight history and severity of weight loss, if any, the focus should be on maximizing oral intake or providing alternate feeding as soon as possible if oral intake is not feasible or is unachievable. Malnutrition is quite common in patients in hospitals and nursing homes.

Approximately 70–80% of malnourished patients currently enter and leave the hospital without healthcare practitioners acting to treat their malnutrition and without the diagnosis appearing on their discharge summary (Lean, 2008).

Factors attributed to malnutrition include anorexia, adjusting to hospitalization, dysphagia, metabolic disorder (e.g., cachexia secondary to cancer), AIDS, malabsorption, gastrointestinal distress, and a delayed response to poor caloric and protein intake.

Research studies indicate that up to 55% of older adults admitted to hospitals suffer from malnutrition. The challenge, therefore, is to prevent weight loss because unplanned severe weight loss correlates with poor nutrition outcome and increases length of stay in the hospital.

Table 1-1 Interpretation of Percentage Weight Change

Interpretation

Weight loss/gain of 1% to 2% in 1 week is significant. Weight loss/gain of > 2% in 1 week is severe.

Time	Significant Weight Loss (%)	Severe Weight Loss (%)
1 week	1–2	> 2
1 month	5	> 5
3 months	7.5	> 7.5
6 months	10	> 10

SKIN INTEGRITY

A pressure ulcer or pressure sore is a localized injury to the skin and/or underlying tissue, usually over a bony prominence, as a result of pressure. Pressure ulcers usually result from an inadequate supply of oxygen and nutrients to the skin's epithelial and supportive tissues. Pressure ulcers are staged to classify the degree of tissue damage observed. (See **Table 1–2**.)

The number of hospital patients with pressure sores, also called decubitus ulcers or bed sores, rose from 280,000 cases in 1993 to 455,000 cases in 2003—a 63% increase—according to data from the Department of Health and Human Services Agency for Healthcare Research and Quality (AHRQ) (Russo & Elixhauser, 2006).

Usually, nurses assess the skin integrity of the patient/resident using the Braden Scale and document it in the medical chart. However, because nutrition plays such a vital role in the healing process, the dietitian must be involved and must address matters relating to wound healing.

The Centers for Medicare and Medicaid Services (CMS) guidelines released on November 12, 2004, stipulate that facilities need to concentrate on residents' risk factors for and prevention of pressure sores, not just the Braden Scale (Beckrich & Aronovitch, 1999).

Risk Factors Associated With Delayed Wound Healing

Immobility and inactivity are primary risk factors for developing pressure ulcers. Malnutrition characterized by protein-calorie deficiency, anemia,

Table 1-2 Stages of Pressure Ulcers

Stages of Pressure Ulcers	Description	Nutrition Consideration
Stage I	Skin is warm to touch. Usually a persistent area of redness in lightly pigmented skin. In darker skin tones, the ulcer may appear with persistent red, blue, or purple hues.	• Ensure adequate caloric and fluid intake. • Recommend 30–35 cal/kg and 0.8–1.1 g protein per kg, more for patients who are malnourished or who have an albumin level < 3.5 mg/dL. • Add MVI to regimen.
Stage II	Partial thickness skin loss involving epidermis, dermis, or both. The ulcer is superficial and presents clinically as an abrasion, blister, or a shallow open ulcer.	• Ensure adequate caloric and fluid intake. • Recommend 30–35 cal/kg. • Recommend 1.1–1.3 g protein/kg, more for patients who are malnourished or who have an albumin level < 3.5 mg/dL. • Add MVI once a day and vitamin C 500 mg once a day to regimen.
Stage III	Full thickness skin loss involving damage to, necrosis of subcutaneous tissue that may extend down to, but not through underlying fascia.	• Ensure adequate caloric and fluid intake. • Recommend 35 cal/kg and 1.3–1.5 g protein/kg. • Add MVI once a day and vitamin C 500 mg per day.
Stage IV	Full thickness skin loss with extensive destruction, tissue necrosis, or damage to muscle, bone, or supporting structures (e.g., tendon, joint capsule).	• Ensure adequate caloric and fluid intake. • Recommend 35 cal/kg. Increase calories if patient is underweight or has had weight loss. • Recommend 1.5–2.0 g protein/kg body weight. • Add MVI once a day, vitamin C 500 mg twice a day. (Zinc is recommended only if there is evidence of zinc deficiency.)

vitamin deficiency, and dehydration is also a major risk factor. Malnutrition impedes healing for both chronic and acute wounds. Dehydration can result in an increase in blood glucose, which slows the healing process. Steroids and anticoagulants can also delay wound healing. Impaired wound healing may occur in patients taking glucocorticoids because these drugs suppress inflammatory cells and collagen synthesis (Ayello & Cuddington, 2004). The use of anticoagulants such as heparin/warfarin has a negative impact on the earliest stage of wound healing.

Patients who are immunocompromised such as older adults, those with cancer, and those with HIV/AIDS have reduced or delayed inflammatory response and may be at risk for infection or wound compromise. It is important that you assess for adequate calorie, protein, and fluid intake to aid wound healing.

Several randomized controlled trials have concluded that vitamin C, zinc, and arginine improve the rate of pressure ulcer healing (Desneves, Todorovic, Cassar, & Crowe, 2005). Clinical trials have demonstrated an improvement in healing rates with enhanced enteral formulas containing zinc, arginine, and vitamin C. Zinc is especially useful when there is a decrease in serum albumin.

Preventing Pressure Ulcers

The goal for pressure ulcers should be zero occurrences. Pressure ulcer prevention strategies should include the following six key elements:

- Conduct a pressure ulcer admission assessment for all patients.
- Reassess risk for all patients daily.
- Inspect skin daily.
- Manage moisture.
- Optimize nutrition and hydration.
- Minimize pressure. (Duncan, 2007)

Pressure ulcers are costly and painful and can be fatal if not treated aggressively. Preventing pressure ulcers help to save healthcare dollars.

GASTROINTESTINAL REVIEW

The gastrointestinal review looks at all factors involving the gastrointestinal (GI) tract and its impact on nutritional status.

Nausea and Vomiting

Nausea is an uneasiness of the stomach that often accompanies the urge to vomit, but doesn't always lead to vomiting. Vomiting, or emesis, can be caused by gastroparesis, as in uncontrolled diabetes, chemotherapy in cancer patients, food allergies, viral infection, or medications.

Investigate the nature of the emesis. Does the emesis consist of partially or fully digested food? Is it coffee ground in color, or is there blood? Coffee-ground emesis is indicative of gastrointestinal bleeding, which could cause a decrease in hemoglobin and hematocrit. It results from blood that has been in the stomach for a period of time, which indicates a slow bleed. An active GI bleed is indicated by bloody emesis.

It is also important to know when the vomiting occurs. Is it after meals? If so, how long after the meal does it occur? After which foods are consumed does the vomiting occur? This information is crucial to the nutrition intervention. Food elimination may be necessary if vomiting occurs consistently with some foods. Also consider that gastric tumor may cause emesis of undigested food. Emesis that is yellow or green may suggest the presence of bile, which could indicate gallbladder disease.

Nutritional Implications and Intervention

Persistent nausea and vomiting have the potential for anorexia with subsequent weight loss and dehydration. Bloody emesis can cause anemia, causing weakness and dizziness with increased risk for falls, especially in older adults. Vomiting decreases potassium and sodium levels as well. It is not unusual for a patient to report "being afraid to eat" lest he starts vomiting. Fluids should be encouraged and high-potassium foods given to prevent electrolyte imbalance. You must investigate the cause of the vomiting and address it. The diet should be low in fiber and fat. A promotility drug or other antiemetic medication is usually given to increase gastric emptying.

Stools and Diarrhea

Diarrhea is defined as the frequent passage of liquid stools greater than three per day for two consecutive days that may or may not be associated with a pathologic state. Some patients experience diarrhea with the use of antibiotics, and this may last for the duration of the antibiotic therapy. Diarrhea can also be caused by viral gastroenteritis; food poisoning;

malabsorption syndrome, which includes lactose intolerance, gluten malabsorption, inflammatory bowel disease—Crohn's disease, ulcerative colitis, and irritable bowel syndrome. Chemotherapy and laxatives containing magnesium are also associated with diarrhea.

Upper gastrointestinal (GI) bleed may cause dark, tarry stools. Iron supplements, however, may cause the stool to be dark as well, so a guaiac test is usually performed to determine the presence of blood. Stool sample is smeared on a card to test for blood in the stool. A dark red to black tarry appearance of the stool is indicative of a loss of 0.5 mL to 0.75 mL of blood from the upper gastrointestinal tract. Inflammatory bowel disease, stomach ulcers, colitis, and hemorrhoids may cause GI bleed.

Meat consumption prior to a stool test can give a false-positive test because of the presence of hemoglobin and myoglobin in the meat. Aspirin, alcohol, and excess vitamin C in amounts greater than 500 mg/day may cause a false-negative test (Fischbach, 2003).

Lower gastrointestinal bleed tends to cause frank bleeding, that is, obvious bleeding such as vomiting blood or seeing actual blood in the stools. Clay-colored stools may be indicative of jaundice.

Nutritional Implications and Intervention

You must investigate the cause of the diarrhea. If diarrhea is caused by the presence of *Clostridium difficile* (c-diff), antibiotic therapy is usually initiated.

It is wise to avoid lactose products and apple juice because these can exacerbate diarrhea. If persistent diarrhea is not caused by antibiotics, then antidiarrheal medications should be considered to improve diarrhea to prevent weight loss and ensure nutrient adequacy. Whatever the cause of the diarrhea, adequate fluids and electrolytes must be maintained to prevent dehydration and electrolyte imbalance. Oral rehydration solutions are used frequently to ensure electrolyte balance.

A variety of studies have found probiotic consumption to be useful in the treatment of many types of diarrhea, including antibiotic-induced diarrhea in adults. In Finland, the efficacy of *Lactobacillus* GG yogurt in preventing erythromycin-associated diarrhea was studied. Sixteen healthy volunteers were given erythromycin acistrate 400 mg t.i.d. for a week. The volunteers were randomly assigned to one of two groups taking twice daily 125 mL of either *Lactobacillus* GG fermented yogurt or pasteurized regular yogurt as placebo during the drug treatment. Subjects receiving *Lactobacillus*

GG yogurt with erythromycin had less diarrhea than those taking pasteurized yogurt. Other side effects of erythromycin, such as abdominal distress, stomach pain, and flatulence, were less common in the GG yogurt group than in the placebo yogurt group (Siitonen et al., 1990).

Teitelbaum (2005) reports in the *Pediatric Infectious Disease Journal* that probiotics were beneficial in treating infectious diarrhea when co-administered with a variety of antibiotics. The study of 16 healthy volunteers taking erythromycin for 1 week found that co-administration of *Lactobacillus* GG yogurt not only reduced the number of days with diarrhea from 8 to 2 but also decreased associated side effects such as abdominal pain from 39% to 23% (Teitelbaum, 2005).

Stools with a positive guaiac warrant further investigation of the underlying problem, and it should be addressed immediately. Diet should be rich in iron and protein to prevent hypoalbuminemia and anemia.

Constipation and Fecal Impaction

Constipation is the passage of small amounts of hard, dry stools, usually fewer than three times a week. Symptoms of constipation include feeling bloated, uncomfortable, and sluggish. Sudden watery diarrhea in someone who has chronic constipation is usually an indication of a fecal impaction. A fecal impaction is a large mass of dry, hard stool that can develop in the rectum as a result of chronic constipation. This mass may be so hard that it cannot be excreted, so the patient has to be disimpacted. In severe cases, the patient may require hospitalization. Fecal impaction can be fatal.

Contributory Factors

Specific factors contribute to constipation and fecal impaction:

- *Specific diseases/disorders*: Several disorders can cause constipation. These include neurologic disorders such as multiple sclerosis, Parkinson's disease, stroke, and spinal injuries. Metabolic and endocrine conditions including diabetes, underactive or overactive thyroid glands, and hypercalcemia also contribute to constipation.
- *Medications*: Medications that can cause constipation include pain medications (especially narcotics), antacids that contain aluminum and calcium, blood pressure medications (calcium channel blockers), anti-Parkinson drugs, antispasmodics, antidepressants, iron supplements, diuretics, and anticonvulsants.

- *Lack of physical activity.* Lack of physical activity can lead to constipation. Bedridden patients with stroke, dementia, or cerebral palsy are at high risk. The frequent use of laxatives for elimination over time can lead to loss of bowel function, causing chronic constipation.
- *Caffeine and alcohol.* Alcohol and liquids containing caffeine, such as coffee and cola drinks, have a diuretic effect and can increase the risk for dehydration and subsequent constipation.

Nutritional Implications and Intervention

Constipation causes bloating and discomfort and affects the patient's appetite. The risk of constipation can be reduced by encouraging the patient to increase fluid intake, gradually introduce fiber in the diet, and avoid excessive intake of banana, which can promote constipation. Encourage patients to limit intake of caffeine-containing beverages and increase physical activity, including range of motion for those who are bedridden.

The Prevalence of Enteral/Parenteral Nutrition (Nutrition Support)

Enteral Nutrition

If a patient's oral intake is suboptimal, proper documentation such as calorie count and/or food record of oral intake with percentages consumed should be in place to support the need for alternate feeding. If the patient is unable to make decisions about alternate feeding, contact the family to make the decision. In the absence of family involvement, the matter should be referred to the ethics committee of the facility for a decision to be made.

Enteral nutrition is administered into the gastrointestinal tract via percutaneous endoscopic gastrostomy (PEG), a nasogastric tube (NGT), percutaneous endoscopic jejunostomy (PEJ), or a orogastric tube (OGT).

Indications for early enteral nutrition include the following:

- Major head injuries, torso or abdominal trauma
- Major upper GI surgery that precludes oral intake for > 5 days
- Second- or third-degree burns over more than 20% of the body
- Chronical malnourishment in patients anticipated to be without oral intake for > 5 days

Enteral nutrition support is contraindicated in the following situations:
- When aggressive therapy is not warranted—poor prognosis
- When there is intractable vomiting or diarrhea
- Intestinal obstruction, peritonitis, short bowel syndrome with 75% or more resection of the small intestine and ileus
- When there is high output proximal fistula
- When a patient has severe acute pancreatitis

The caloric and protein needs of the patient are based on his or her medical condition. Formulas are designed to meet specific needs, for example, formula containing reduced carbohydrate for patients with diabetes, branched chain amino acids for patients with liver failure, and reduced water for patients with pulmonary conditions. Specialized formulas containing extra protein and calories, glutamine, arginine, and zinc are used for the critically ill patient. Adequate calories should be provided so that protein is not used for energy.

A patient new to tube feeding should start feeding at a lower rate, for example, 20–40 mL/hour. Calorically dense formulas such as those offering 1.5–2.0 cal/mL should start at a much lower rate of 10–15 mL/hr. Feeding should be gradually advanced in small increments every 8–12 hours until actual caloric needs are met in those patients who are hemodynamically stable. Feeding for the unstable patients should be advanced as can be tolerated.

Complications of Enteral Nutrition Following are the common complications of enteral nutrition:

- *Diarrhea*: Diarrhea and vomiting are associated with too rapid an infusion rate during feeding. Diarrhea can also be the result of intestinal atrophy; medications such as antibiotics, laxatives, or sorbitol-containing meds; or the presence of *Clostridium difficile* bacteria. Poor handling of formula can introduce bacteria as well. A hypertonic formula and hypoalbuminemia are also associated with diarrhea.
- *Constipation*: Constipation while on enteral nutrition can be attributed to lack of activity, inadequate fluids and fiber, and use of pain medications and narcotics.
- *Refeeding syndrome*: Refeeding syndrome can occur if the malnourished patient is fed too aggressively. Refeeding syndrome is charac-

terized by acute drops in the plasma levels of phosphorus, potassium, and magnesium. It may involve anemia, respiratory distress, tetany, and severe or fatal cardiac arrythmias. Monitoring of electrolytes, fluid input/output, glucose, and daily weights is important in preventing refeeding syndrome.

- *Aspiration*: A misplaced tube can cause aspiration. Patients receiving tube feeding may experience apirations evidenced by repeated pneumonia with an increase in temperature. A jejunostomy tube may be considered as an alternate route for feeding, though there is never an absolute lack of risk of aspiration. Other contributory factors to aspiration include decreased intestinal motility and gastric emptying. It is important that the head of the bed be elevated at a 45° angle during feeding to prevent aspiration.

- *Dehydration*: Dehydration in patients receiving enteral nutrition is associated with a hypertonic formula without sufficient free water. Excessive protein intake and hyperglycemia also can cause dehydration. Fluid needs are estimated at 1 mL/cal. You must calculate the water content of the formula and the water used for medications, and then determine free water flushes to meet the fluid needs of the patient. If there is evidence of constipation, increase fluids; however, be sure to monitor electrolytes to ensure that there is no hypervolemia (fluid overload).

- *Overhydration*: Overhydration of patients receiving enteral nutrition can lead to hyponatremia, or low serum sodium. Symptoms of hyponatremia include fatigue, lethargy, confusion, seizures, decreased consciousness, or coma. Reducing fluid intake can correct the sodium level.

- *High gastric residual volume*: Gastric residual volume is used as an indicator of the patient's tolerance for enteral feeding. Residuals should be less than 200 mL. If there is a high residual volume in the patient who is tube fed, take the following actions:
  1. Switch to a low-fat, low-fiber formula or diet if the patient is being fed orally as well.
  2. Administer the solution at room temperature.
  3. Consider adding Reglan (metoclopramide) for increased gastric emptying.
  4. Reduce tube feeding rate.

5. Consider a proton pump inhibitor to improve the integrity of the gastrointestinal tract; examples include Protonix (pantoprazole), Prevacid (lansoprozole), Prilosec (omeprazole), Nexium (esomeprazole magnesium).

6. Tighten glycemic control in the diabetic patient to glucose < 200 mg/dL.

7. Do not stop feeding, but repeat residuals in 4 hours.

8. If no improvement occurs, consider total parenteral nutrition (TPN).

Monitor patients who are receiving enteral nutrition carefully for electrolyte balance. Dilantin (phenytoin), an anticonvulsant, should be given 2 hours before or after tube feeding to increase bioavailability of the drug.

Parenteral Nutrition

Parenteral nutrition is usually administered into the veins. Peripheral parenteral nutrition (PPN) is administered into the veins of the arm, whereas total parenteral nutrition (TPN) is administered into the superior or inferior vena cava or the jugular vein. TPN is also called IVH, intravenous hyperalimentation.

Medicare guidelines stipulate that daily TPN be considered reasonable and necessary for a patient with severe pathology of the alimentary tract that does not allow absorption of sufficient nutrients to maintain weight and strength commensurate with the patient's general condition.

Qualifications for Parenteral Nutrition Conditions that qualify for parenteral nutrition include the following:

- A condition involving the small intestine and/or its exocrine glands that significantly impairs the absorption of nutrients.
- Disease of the stomach and/or intestine which is a motility disorder and impairs the ability of nutrients to be absorbed through the GI system The gut does not work.
- Need for nothing by mouth (NPO) status longer than 7 days, or few days if the patient presents with high nutrition risk.
- Nutritional needs that are greater than the amount of nutrients that can be delivered enterally.

Contraindications for Parenteral Nutrition Parenteral nutrition should not be used in the following situations:

- When there is a functioning GI tract
- When prognosis is poor
- In mild to moderate nutrition risk patients with short-term NPO status

Factors to consider for parenteral nutrition are caloric, fluid, protein, carbohydrate, fat, vitamin, mineral, and electrolyte needs of the patient.

Components of Parenteral Nutrition
- *Carbohydrate:* In the form of dextrose. Dextrose concentrations vary from 10% to 70%. Dextrose is calculated at 3.4 cal/g.
- *Protein:* Amino acids (AA) are available in 3% to 10% solutions. AA is calculated at 4 cal/g.
- *Lipids:* Available in 10–20% solutions. Ten percent lipids are calculated at 1.1 cal/mL and, 20% lipids at 2 cal/mL.
- *Electrolytes:* Provided as part of the general solutions to meet requirements. Amounts vary according to individual patient needs.
- *Vitamins and minerals:* Daily maintenance dosage given in standard solutions. May be adjusted to meet patient needs.
- *Trace elements:* Maintenance dosage provided in standard solutions.
- *Medications:* Insulin may be added to the solution for blood glucose control.

Calculating Parenteral Nutrition Formulas
1. *Calculate caloric needs.* Using the sample patient described in the preceding table, the caloric requirement is 1860 cal /day (30 cal/kg; $30 \times 62 = 1860$ calories).
2. *Determine protein needs.* Assuming that the patient is moderately ill, provide 1.2 g/kg to 1.5 g/kg. Protein needs would therefore be 74–93 g/day.
3. *Determine if the solution meets the needs of the patient.* First, find the volume of solution provided to the patient. Infusion for this patient begins at 18:00 hours (6 pm) and runs until 10:00 hours (10 am) at 84 mL/hr providing 1344 mL of solution over 16 hours. At 10:10 am the rate was reduced to 63 mL/hr to run for 8 hours providing 504 mL.

Sample Parenteral Nutrition Description

Patient: Jane Doe

Age: 64 years

Sex: Female

Height: 64.0 inches

Weight: 62 kg

Medication Description

Large Volumes	Dose	Dose Quantity	Rate Frequency	Next Time
Dextrose 40%	400 g	1 ea	84 mL/hr IV	10/31/08 18:00 hrs
Freamine III 10% 1000 mL	100 g	1 ea		
Sodium chloride 23.4% 30 mL	154 mEq	1.2833 ea	63 mL/hr Administer at 10 am daily and infuse over 8 hours	11/1/08 10:00 hrs
Potassium acetate 40 mEq/20 mL INJ	38 mEq	0.95 ea		
Calcium gluconate 10% 10 mL INJ	18.6047 mEq	4 ea		
Magnesium sulfate 50% 2 mL INJ	12.8 mEq	1.58 ea		
Multi trace elements 5 1 mL	1 mL	1 ea		
MVI12 10 mL INJ	10 mL	1 ea		
Potassium phosphate 3 mmo/mL 5mL	44 mEq	2 ea		
Potassium chloride 40 mEq/20 mL INJ	60 mEq	1.5 ea		
Insulin human reg 100 U/mL (LVP)	30 U	0.3 mL		
Lipid 10% 500 mL	500 mL	1 ea		

Also contains phosphate 20 mEq, sodium 10 mEq, and acetate 89 mEq

Total run time is 24 hours providing 1848 mL of solution. Note well that the constituents of the solution indicated on the TPN description are per 1000 mL (1 liter) of solution.

Calculate:

Calories from dextrose: $1.848 \text{ L} \times 400 \times 3.4 = 2513$ cal

Calories from fat: $1.848 \text{ L} \times 500 \times 1.1 = 1016$ cal

Total non-protein cal $= 3529$ cal

Total protein $1.848 \text{ L} \times 100 = 185$ g

Calories from protein (freamine) $1.848 \text{ L} \times 100 \times 4 = 739$ cal

The solution above provides calories and protein in excess of required amounts. Unlike enteral nutrition formula, TPN usually begins at a high rate and decreases gradually. Monitor patient for weight gain. Insulin is provided to reduce the risk of hyperglycemia.

Nutritional Implications and Intervention Careful documentation must be in place to support the need for parenteral nutrition (PN). Review such documentation periodically for possible weaning and transitioning to oral or enteral nutrition.

A patient who is placed on PN who has been without nutrition for some time is at risk for **refeeding syndrome**. To minimize the risk of refeeding syndrome in PN patients, administer PN at one half the total calories and increase nutritional intake gradually to estimated nutritional requirements.

The National Institute for Clinical Excellence (NICE) recently recommended that parenteral nutrition should be limited to a maximum of 50% of the calculated requirements for the first 48 hours after initiation.

Hyperglycemia is associated with the initiation of PN and sometimes requires the use of insulin to control high blood glucose especially in patients who have diabetes or who experience sepsis. Blood glucose should be monitored frequently.

There is an increased risk for sepsis in patients receiving PN because the gut is not being used. There is also the risk of overfeeding critically ill patients, consequences of which can be fatal. Excessive carbohydrate infusion can result in hypercapnia, which increases the work of the lungs and potentially prolongs the need for mechanical ventilation. Overfeeding can also lead to hyperglycemia and an accumulation of fat in the liver. Severe hyperglycemia results in profound dehydration.

Excessive protein can lead to azotemia, hypertonic dehydration, and metabolic acidosis if the kidneys are unable to properly adjust urea excretion or acid–base balance. Hypertriglyceridemia and fat overload can occur as a result of excessive fat infusion. Monitor blood triglycerides closely. Respiratory distress, coagulopathies, and abnormal liver function tests are the primary manifestations of fat overload (Klein, Stanek, & Wiles 1998). The energy goal is based on the patient's actual weight and 25–30 cal/kg is recommended. The protein recommendation ranges from 1.5–2.0 g/kg body weight depending on the severity of illness. Use the ideal body weight to determine caloric and protein requirements in obese patients.

CARDIOVASCULAR REVIEW

The cardiovascular review takes into consideration the presence of a cerebral vascular accident (CVA) or stroke, congestive heart failure (CHF) or pleural effusion, angina, myocardial infarction (heart attack), hypertension, and obesity. If the patient presents with diabetes, the risk of coronary artery disease is increased. Diabetes causes an increase in triglycerides and a decrease in high-density lipoprotein (HDL). In most cases, once blood glucose is controlled and weight is decreased, triglycerides improve drastically even without medication.

Cerebral Vascular Accident

Cerebral vascular accidents (CVAs), commonly known as stroke, usually occur as a result of uncontrolled hypertension. In most cases, CVAs affect the patient's swallowing ability, speech, and ability to feed himself or herself. Patients experience an overall decline in activities of daily living (ADLs). The stroke patient is at increased risk for weight loss resulting from decline in swallowing and feeding skills. Encourage patients to use adaptive feeding devices to attain some level of independent feeding. Proper positioning is extremely important. The patient should be positioned at or close to a 90° angle as much as possible. The speech therapist determines the consistency of fluids and solids because most patients who have suffered a stroke are dysphagic.

If a patient is on a modified consistency, for example, a pureed diet, consult the speech pathologist before advancing the diet, even if the patient shows improvement in chewing and/or swallowing skills.

A diet low in sodium is usually recommended to help control hypertension. Other complications with CVA include pressure sores and contractures resulting from immobility.

Congestive Heart Failure

Congestive heart failure (CHF) occurs when the heart loses its ability to act as a pump. Some precipitating causes are pulmonary embolism, infection, anemia, myocarditis, arrythmias, and myocardial infarction.

Some symptoms of heart failure are shortness of breath; fatigue or weakness; persistent coughing or wheezing; swelling of the legs, ankles, and feet; third spacing fluid accumulation in the abdomen; lack of appetite; confused thinking; and increased or irregular heartbeat.

Angina and Myocardial Infarction

Heart disease remains the number one killer in the United States. Angina or chest pain occurs when the supply of oxygen to the heart becomes low. Angina is usually a precipitating factor of a heart attack, though not all chest pains are related to a heart condition. If blood flow to the heart is reduced as a result of buildup of plaque, primarily cholesterol along the artery (atherosclerosis), heart cells can die, resulting in a heart attack.

Patients who have diabetes or HIV/AIDS are at increased risk for heart disease. Most patients with type 2 diabetes present with increased triglycerides and decreased HDL. Medications such as Kaletra (lopinavir, ritovavir) used to treat HIV/AIDS patients may cause an increase in triglycerides. Increased triglycerides alone are not a risk factor for heart disease, but suggests to the clinician that there is an increased intake of carbohydrates, especially simple carbohydrates. Increased alcohol intake can also cause an increase in triglycerides. Risk factors for coronary heart disease include age, hereditary factors, overweight, smoking, high blood pressure, and sedentary lifestyle.

Increased homocysteine, an amino acid, in the blood is also associated with coronary heart disease. Folic acid and vitamin B_{12} are usually given to reduce homocysteine levels, but no studies prove that an individual can reduce his or her risk of coronary heart disease by taking these supplements (National Institutes of Health, 2005).

The lipid profile of the patient is the most important blood test for risk assessment. C-reactive protein (CRP), a substance produced in the liver, when elevated has been shown to be associated with an increased risk of heart disease. However, most physicians will not order this test unless the lipids associated with heart disease are also elevated, such as low-density lipoprotein (LDL), total cholesterol, and triglycerides, and also if high-density lipoprotein (HDL) is reduced. CRP levels less than 1 mg/L are considered low risk for a cardiovascular event in the next 10 years. Depending on medical history and other factors, a person having a CRP of 1–3 mg/L could have up to a 20% risk of having a heart attack in the next decade. Those with CRP levels of 3 mg/L or more per liter have the highest risk (National Institutes of Health, 2005).

Lowering high blood pressure and other lifestyle changes can help reduce CRP and improve overall cardiovascular health.

Hypertension

Hypertension is defined as blood pressure greater than 140/90 mmHg. Smoking, high cholesterol, obesity, and diabetes increase the risk of hypertension. The incidence of high blood pressure increases with age, but is today seen in children and adolescents, especially those who are overweight. Uncontrolled hypertension can affect the blood vessels, causing them to become thicker and less elastic, and blood clots can form and stick to the vessel walls. If a clot becomes dislodged, it can enter the bloodstream and do serious damage to various organs.

Prolonged high blood pressure can cause poor blood flow to the heart muscle, so the muscle cannot get the oxygen it needs, thereby causing ischemia. Over time, the heart grows larger; heart enlargement is one of the causes of cardiovascular disease. Besides affecting the heart and blood vessels, prolonged high blood pressure can affect the brain, as in stroke; the kidneys, reducing blood flow and weakening them; and can cause blood vessel constriction, tiny bleeding, and deposits of fat in the eyes. These changes in the eye result in worsening vision and loss of sight.

Obesity

There is a direct association between abdominal obesity and the risk of coronary heart disease. The Framingham Heart Study confirms that obesity is strongly predictive of CHD. Risk for CVD is particularly raised when abdominal obesity is present. Abdominal obesity is defined by a waist circumference greater than 102 cm (40 inches), in men, or 88 cm (35 inches) in women (National Cholesterol Education Program, Third Report, 2009). Encourage the individuals to make lifestyle changes to reduce weight and subsequent risk of heart disease.

Medications Used to Treat Heart Failure

Several types of drugs have been used and are proven useful in the treatment of heart failure. These include angiotensin-converting enzyme (ACE) inhibitors such as Vasotec (enalapril), lisinopril, and captopril; and angiotensin II receptor blockers (ARBs), which include losartan and Diovan (valsartan). These drugs decrease the workload of the heart. Digoxin, also referred to as digitalis, increases the strength of the heart muscle contractions and tends to slow the heartbeat. Beta blockers such as Coreg (carvedilol), Lopressor (metoprolol tartrate) and Zebeta (bisoprolol fumarate) also slow the heart rate.

Diuretics, for example, Furosemide (Lasix) and Spironolactone (Aldactone), are used to reduce fluid retention in patients with congestive heart failure. Lasix is potassium wasting, causing a decrease in serum potassium. Unlike Lasix, Aldactone is primarily potassium sparing. Aldactone prevents salt retention because it inhibits the production of aldosterone known to increase blood pressure.

Nutritional Implications and Intervention

Because of altered fluid status in the patient with congestive heart failure, weight must be interpreted with caution. The patient's oral intake, diet, and weight history provide needed information to determine caloric needs.

Fluid and electrolyte status must be monitored closely. Lasix can cause an increase in blood glucose (Pronsky, 1997). Renal function and potassium levels should be monitored regularly. Potassium supplements are usually given when potassium level drops significantly low. Spironolactone (Aldactone), on the other hand, can raise the level of potassium in the blood to dangerous levels, at which time a potassium-lowering drug such as Kayexalate (sodium polystyrene) may be given to improve hyperkalemia. High potassium can affect heart function. Diarrhea usually occurs with Kayexalate; fluids should therefore be monitored to prevent dehydration.

It is not unusual for a patient with CHF to develop cardiac cachexia, characterized by a marked loss of adipose tissue and lean body mass. Anorexia, depression, nausea and vomiting, and difficulty breathing because of pulmonary edema are some of the precipitating factors in the development of cardiac cachexia.

Restricted activity and a diet low in sodium are usually recommended for the patient with CHF. Fluid restriction may be necessary to help control retention of fluid.

The initial intervention for the patient who presents with the risk factors of coronary heart disease is lifestyle changes—weight loss for overweight patients, smoking cessation, a diet low in fat and cholesterol, reduced intake of simple carbohydrates to control hypertriglyceridemia, good glucose control for patients with diabetes, and increased physical activity. These all help to reduce low-density lipoprotein (LDL) and increase high-density lipoprotein (HDL). A low-sodium diet is also recommended to help control hypertension. The goal is to achieve and maintain a blood pressure of less than 130/80 mmHg. Medications, such as those used for patients with congestive heart failure, are also used to control high blood pressure.

Soluble fiber found in oats, legumes, fruits, and psyllium helps to lower cholesterol and LDL. Niacin is also used with good effect but can cause increased bleeding when used in combination with anticoagulants. Niacin should not be used in patients with kidney problems.

Aspirin or other anticoagulants such as Coumadin (warfarin) are added to prevent blood clots. Monitor the patient's platelets and International Normalized Ratio (INR) regularly when on anticoagulants to ensure that there is no bleeding.

For patients with diabetes, check their lipid profile one to two times a year. It is also important that there be pre-prandial and postprandial readings to determine efficacy of medication and diet regimen. Check hemoglobin AIC two to four times a year as part of the patient's scheduled medical visit (Joslin Diabetes Center, 2009).

PSYCHIATRIC REVIEW

The psychiatric review of the patient takes into consideration the patient's mental status including his level of consciousness; orientation to place, person, and time; impaired or unimpaired memory; decision-making skills; communication skills; presence of hallucination and illusion; and psychomotor behavior. Psychomotor behavior looks at whether the patient resists care, medication, or food; exhibits inappropriate or disruptive behavior such as smearing or throwing feces; is self-abusive; or displays sexual behavior, screaming, disrobing in public, noisiness, or disruptive sounds.

Some patients might not display disruptive behavior but may have mood issues. They may be sad or worried most of the time; may have reduced social interaction, self-depreciation, repetitive physical movements, repetitive physical complaints, fearfulness, paranoia, insomnia, persistent anger with others; and others cry a lot. Diagnoses that suggest psychosis include anxiety disorder, depression, and bipolar disorder.

Nutritional Implications and Intervention

All of the psychiatric situations mentioned have some impact on the patient's nutritional status. Medications used for psychosis and their interaction with nutrition are discussed later in this chapter. Some antidepressants such as Prozac (fluoxetine) and Luvox (fluvoxamine meleate) may cause constipation, thereby increasing the patient's need for extra fluids. Patients who take lithium to treat manic depressive disorder should maintain a consistent intake of sodium to stabilize the drug level because low sodium intake can cause delay in the excretion of lithium from the body, which might result in lithium toxicity. Other conditions that can lower sodium and cause a buildup of lithium include heavy sweating, fever, vomiting, diarrhea, and use of diuretics. Patients taking lithium should have adequate fluid intake to reduce toxicity of the drug.

Abilify (aripiprazole) used to treat schizophrenia and acute manic bipolar disorder has been associated with increased blood sugar.

Those patients with dementia including Alzheimer's disease tend to
wander a lot and hardly ever sit to eat a meal. They are usually agitated
and restless. Frequent wandering may increase energy needs as much as
1600 calories or more/day. Patient may make inappropriate food choices,
forget to eat, or have problem recalling if they have eaten. These patients
are at risk for weight loss and should be closely monitored. Offer small
frequent meals one plate at a time—finger foods are best.

Some patients are paranoid, thinking that someone is trying to kill
them by poisoning their food, so they refuse to eat. They do better with
packaged and canned foods, which should be opened in their presence.
Encouragement and support are always needed to ensure desirable outcomes for psychotic patients. A thorough review of the patient's mental
status is important so that you can plan appropriately for the interview
and intervention.

INFECTIOUS DISEASES

Infectious diseases include hepatitis A, B, and C; HIV/AIDS; tuberculosis, malaria, food-borne illnesses, bacterial meningitis, bacterial pneumonia, gastroenteritis, urinary tract infection, typhoid fever, dysentery, and
cholera to name a few.

This section focuses on some of the more common infectious diseases
seen in acute and long-term care, namely, hepatitis A, B, and C; HIV/
AIDS; urinary tract infection; tuberculosis; bacterial pneumonia; and
meningitis.

Hepatitis A

Hepatitis A is a liver disease caused by the hepatitis A virus. Hepatitis A is
transmitted by the fecal-oral route and is contracted through contami-
nated drinking water, food, and sewage. Symptoms include anorexia,
nausea, vomiting, abdominal pain, dark urine, and jaundice. Serious complications can occur in patients whose immune system is compromised
such as older adults and very young children.

In 2007, 2,979 acute symptomatic cases of hepatitis A were reported.
The estimated number of new infections was 25,000 (Centers for Disease
Control and Prevention, 2009a).

Hepatitis B

Hepatitis B is a serious disease caused by a virus that attacks the liver. The virus, which is called hepatitis B virus (HBV), can cause lifelong infection, cirrhosis (scarring) of the liver, liver cancer, liver failure, and death.

During the past 10 years, an estimated 60,000–110,000 persons were infected with HBV annually, and 5,000 died from HBV-related disease in the United States (Finelli & Bell, 2008). More than 350 million people worldwide are infected with the hepatitis B virus. An estimated 620,000 persons worldwide die from hepatitis B virus-related liver disease each year (Centers for Disease Control and Prevention, 2009b).

Hepatitis B is a blood-borne disease and is transmitted via intravenous (IV) drug use, sex, and childbirth. Hepatitis B infection is common among healthcare workers.

Signs and symptoms of hepatitis B infection are similar to those of hepatitis A—jaundice, fatigue, abdominal pain, loss of appetite, nausea, vomiting, and joint pain.

According the Centers for Disease Control and Prevention (2009), about 30% of persons have no signs or symptoms.

Hepatitis C

Hepatitis C is a disease of the liver caused by the hepatitis C virus (HCV). It is one of the most common causes of chronic liver disease in the United States today, affecting more than 4 million Americans. At least 80% of patients with acute hepatitis C ultimately develop chronic liver infection, and 20% to 30% develop cirrhosis. Between 1% and 5% of patients may develop liver cancer. Hepatitis C is now the number-one cause for liver transplantation in the United States (National Institutes of Health, 2002).

Symptoms of hepatitis C infection include jaundice, abdominal pain (right upper abdomen), fatigue, loss of appetite, nausea and vomiting, low-grade fever, pale or clay-colored stools, dark urine, generalized itching, and bleeding varices (dilated veins throughout the gastrointestinal tract).

Nutritional Implications and Intervention

The liver is the largest and one of the most versatile organs in the body. Its functions include the following:

- *Carbohydrate metabolism:* The liver stores glucose as glycogen, breaks down glycogen to supply glucose when levels become low, and produces glucose from noncarbohydrate sources such as lactic acid and amino acids.

- *Conversion of amino acids to glucose and the synthesis of non-essential amino acids.*
- *Detoxification of ammonia:* The liver converts ammonia to urea for excretion by the kidneys.
- *Storage of fat-soluble vitamins and some minerals as well as vitamin B$_{12}$.*
- *Synthesis of triglycerides, phospholipids, cholesterol, and bile salts.* Bile is essential for the absorption of the fat-soluble vitamins A, D, E, and K.
- *Removal of bacteria, alcohol, and toxic substances from the blood:* The liver converts toxins to substances that can be excreted from the body.
- *Synthesis of drugs and medications.*

When the liver is damaged its functioning is impaired.

Malnutrition is quite common in patients with chronic liver disease. Factors that contribute to malnutrition include a severely restricted diet, altered taste, portal hypertension, weakness, fatigue, early satiety in the presence of ascites, and malabsorption leading to inadequate intake of calories and protein. Protein-calorie malnutrition (PCM)—a condition of body wasting related to dietary deficiency of calories and protein—is found in 65–90% of patients with advanced liver disease and in almost 100% of candidates for liver transplantation (Henkel & Buchman, 2006).

Patients with hepatitis accompanied by ascites and varices should receive a sodium-restricted diet. In the absence of hepatic encephalopathy, protein should be increased greater than or equal to 1.5 g/kg of body weight. If the patient is experiencing hepatic encephalopathy evidenced by neurologic changes and an increase in ammonia level, a diet providing 0.8–1.0 g/kg is considered adequate because severe restriction of protein may cause further malnutrition.

A high ammonia level in the absence of neurologic changes is not considered hepatic encephalopathy. Most physicians will prescribe lactulose and/or neomycin to treat patients with hepatic encephalopathy. Lactulose causes diarrhea, and therefore fluid and electrolytes should be replenished to avoid dehydration. Branch chain amino acids (BCAA) supplementation may improve hepatic encephalopathy.

Patients with liver disease should be encouraged to avoid substances that are toxic to the liver, including alcohol. Even moderate amounts of alcohol speed up the progression of hepatitis C, and alcohol reduces the effectiveness of treatment.

Liver damage can cause bile to back up in the liver so that it is not available to the small intestine for the digestion of fats. When fat is not absorbed, it is excreted in large amounts in the feces, resulting in steatorrhea. Medium-chain triglycerides (MCTs) can help alleviate this condition.

A low serum albumin level is associated with liver disease because the damaged liver cannot synthesize protein and is therefore not a reliable marker for determining nutritional status. Because of fluid shift as in the presence of edema and ascites, you also cannot use weight to determine caloric needs.

In determining nutritional status in the patient with end-stage liver disease (ESLD), Henkel and Buchman (2006) suggest the use of anthropometry, subjective global assessment (SGA), which looks at weight loss during the previous 6 months, changes in dietary intake, gastrointestinal symptoms, functional capacity, metabolic demands, signs of muscle wasting, and the presence of presacral or pedal edema, and also the use of indirect calorimetry. Hand-grip strength was also considered to be a good predictor of complications in patients with advanced liver disease.

The diet should provide adequate calories and protein to prevent or reduce the risk of protein-calorie malnutrition (PCM). Small frequent meals are advised with a late evening snack to reduce protein breakdown. If oral intake is suboptimal, enteral nutrition should be initiated.

HIV/AIDS

HIV (human immunodeficiency virus) is a virus that attacks the body's immune system. The immune system protects the body from infections and diseases.

The Centers for Disease Control and Prevention now estimates that 1.1 million adults and adolescents (prevalence rate: 447.8 per 100,000 population) were living with diagnosed or undiagnosed HIV infection in the United States at the end of 2006. The majority of those living with

HIV were nonwhite (65.4%), and nearly half (48.1%) were men who have sex with men (MSM). The HIV prevalence rates for blacks (1,715.1 per 100,000) and Hispanics (585.3 per 100,000) were, respectively, 7.6 and 2.6 times the rate for whites (224.3 per 100,000; Morbidity and Morality Weekly Report, 2008). An estimated 55,000–58,500 new HIV infections occur in the United States each year (CDC, 2008).

AIDS is the late stage of the HIV infection in which the patient's CD4 cell count falls below 200 or the patient develops serious AIDS-defining diseases including but not limited to wasting syndrome, toxoplasmosis, recurrent pneumonia, esophageal candidiasis, Kaposi's sarcoma, *Mycobacterium avium* complex (MAC), tuberculosis, herpetic ulcers, and progressive multifocal leukoencephalopathy.

A patient may have HIV for a number of years before being diagnosed. Patients may present with flu-like symptoms, headache, cough, diarrhea, swollen glands, lack of energy, loss of appetite, weight loss, fever, sweats, repeated yeast infections, skin rashes, pelvic and abdominal cramps, sores in the mouth or on certain parts of the body, or short-term memory and/or vision loss.

Urinary Tract Infection

Urinary tract infection can occur anywhere along the urinary tract and is usually caused by bacteria from the anus entering the urethra and then the bladder, which leads to inflammation and infection in the lower urinary tract.

Symptoms of a urinary tract infection include pressure in the lower pelvis, pain or burning with urination, frequent or urgent need to urinate, cloudy urine, bloody urine, and foul or strong urine odor.

Pulmonary Tuberculosis

Pulmonary tuberculosis (TB) is a contagious bacterial infection caused by Mycobacterium tuberculosis (M. tuberculosis). The lungs are primarily involved, but the infection can spread to other organs.

Individuals with immune system damage caused by AIDS have a higher risk of developing active tuberculosis—either from new exposure to TB or reactivation of dormant mycobacteria. Symptoms include cough, mild fever, fatigue, unintentional weight loss, hemoptysis, night sweats, and phlegm-producing cough.

Treatment for TB includes rifampin, which can cause a significant increase in uric acid. An increase in uric acid can lead to gouty arthritis.

Pneumonia

Pneumonia is a common illness that affects millions of people each year in the United States. Pneumonia is an inflammation of the lungs caused by an infection. Bacterial pneumonias tend to be the most serious and the most common cause of pneumonia in adults. The most common pneumonia-causing bacterium in adults is Streptococcus pneumoniae (pneumococcus). The main symptoms of pneumonia are cough with greenish or yellow mucus, bloody sputum, fever, sharp or stabbing chest pain worsened by deep breathing or coughing, rapid shallow breathing, and shortness of breath. Other symptoms include headache, loss of appetite, excessive fatigue, and confusion in older people.

Nutritional Implications and Intervention

Most infectious diseases are accompanied by weight loss, increased temperature, anorexia, increased sweat, fatigue, increased risk for dehydration, and shortness of breath as in the case of pneumonia.

Antibiotics are usually administered to treat many infectious diseases, which oftentimes increase the need for more fluids and electrolytes because the patient may experience diarrhea with fluid and electrolyte imbalance.

Pay special attention to adequate nutrition and fluid intake in patients with infectious diseases. High-potassium foods such as fruit juices and banana are recommended for electrolyte replacement. Weight loss is common; therefore the diet should be adequate to meet calorie and protein needs. Small frequent meals are recommended to correct anorexia and fatigue. The patient may also require a nutritional supplement to meet dietary needs if meal intake is inadequate.

Patients treated with highly active antiretroviral therapy (HAART) for the management of HIV/AIDS should be carefully monitored for risk factors of CHD caused by some medications; for example, Kaletra (lopinavir, ritonavir) is known to cause hyperlipidemia. Other medications induce hepatotoxicity, osteopenia/osteoporosis/osteonecrosis, insulin resistance, and hypertension. Anemia is common in patients with HIV/ AIDS; Procrit (epoetin alfa) and ferrous sulphate are usually given to improve this condition.

If the patient presents with oral thrush, modify the diet to allow for easy swallowing.

MUSCULOSKELETAL REVIEW

The musculoskeletal review looks at the body's network of tissues and muscles that are responsible for both voluntary and involuntary movements. Symptoms of decline in the functions of the musculoskeletal system include loss of subcutaneous fat, muscle wasting, edema, painful or swollen joints, and progressive weakness of the muscles. Bow legs, knock knees, and pigeon chest may be a result of protein-energy deficiency and poor intake of vitamins D and C and calcium.

Muscular dystrophy is a disorder of the musculoskeletal system. According to the National Institute of Neurological Disorder and Stroke (2009), muscular dystrophy is characterized by progressive weakness and degeneration of the skeletal muscles that control movement. Medical treatment for muscular dystrophy includes corticosteroids to slow muscle degeneration, anticonvulsants to control seizure and some muscle activity, immunosuppressants to delay dying of muscle cells, and antibiotics to fight respiratory infections. Occupational therapy, physical therapy, and assistive technology are also used in the care of patients with muscular dystrophy.

Nutritional Implications and Intervention

Because the patient's physical movement is compromised, there is an increased risk for overweight, blood clots, calcium deficiency, constipation, and increased blood sugar secondary to use of steroids in patients predisposed to diabetes. Anticonvulsant medications can also contribute to constipation.

The diet should provide adequate calories to maintain normal weight and should also be high in calcium and vitamin D for bone health. In cases where blood thinners are administered to prevent blood clots, monitor the patient for any signs or symptoms of gastrointestinal bleed. Adequate fluids and fiber should be provided to prevent or aid in relieving constipation.

PSYCHOSOCIAL REVIEW

Psychosocial data give information regarding the patient's economic status, occupation, education level, and mental status. This information proves helpful in formulating questions for the interview process. For example, a patient who is undomiciled (homeless) cannot follow a strict diet order; diet teaching must therefore be short and simple with no more than two objectives.

It is important to ascertain patients' food security, which is access to sufficient food at all times for an active and healthy lifestyle; and food insecurity, which is limited or uncertain availability of nutritionally adequate and safe food. Living and shopping arrangements, and availability of a cooking range, refrigerator, and food storage area are critical components that must be included in the psychosocial review of the patient. If the patient has limited access to food, refer the patient to a social worker, who can assist the patient in accessing community resources.

Determining the patient's education level is crucial for the interview. Never assume a patient who has a bachelor's or master's degree is knowledgeable in the area of nutrition and dietetics. As the expert in nutrition, you must ask all the relevant questions needed to complete the assessment thoroughly. Questions may include asking the patient about his or her medical condition and which foods may exacerbate or help improve the outcome. See Chapter 2 for more details.

PULMONARY REVIEW

Gas exchange is the major function of the pulmonary system. The lungs enable the body to obtain oxygen to meet its cellular and metabolic demands and remove the carbon dioxide produced by these processes (Mahan & Escott-Stump, 2008).

There is a strong correlation between malnutrition and pulmonary disease. Malnutrition may impair lung function. Low protein levels resulting from malnutrition contribute to the development of pulmonary edema. When hemoglobin levels are low because of anemia, less oxygen is carried by the blood, resulting in weakness, fatigue, and possibly death. The malnourished patient with lung disease is at risk for developing respiratory infections.

Asthma, bronchitis, and emphysema are collectively known as nonspecific lung diseases. Chronic obstructive pulmonary disease (COPD) is a slowly progressive disease of the airways characterized by a gradual loss of lung function resulting from chronic bronchitis, emphysema, or both. Cigarette smoking is the most important risk factor.

Nutrition Implications and Intervention

Epidemiologic studies indicate that malnourished patients with COPD have a worse prognosis than those who are well nourished. Weight loss in the patient with COPD is caused by the increased work of breathing, frequent recurrent respiratory infections, chronic sputum production, and frequent coughing. Shortness of breath and fatigue can interfere with the patient's ability to prepare and consume meals.

Breathing requires more energy for people with chronic obstructive pulmonary disease (COPD). The muscles used in breathing might require 10 times more calories than those of a person without COPD; hence, the diet must provide adequate calories to meet the increased caloric needs: 30–35 cal/kg is usually recommended for maintenance and 45 cal/kg for anabolism or maintenance during catabolic state.

It is important to monitor biochemical data for any signs of anemia and hypoalbuminemia because these factors can affect the nutritional outcome of the patient with COPD. In the presence of pulmonary edema, sodium should be restricted. Anemia, if present, should be treated aggressively with medication and/or injections such as Aranesp (darbepoetin alfa) or Procrit (epoetin alfa) to enhance good nutritional outcome. The diet should be balanced to provide adequate protein of high biological value and other iron-rich foods. For patients who are on a mechanical ventilator, take care not to overfeed them because this will impede weaning as a result of increased respiratory quotient (RQ—the ratio of carbon dioxide produced to oxygen consumed) and excessive carbon dioxide.

BIOCHEMICAL DATA REVIEW

This section looks at the biochemical data you can use to further assess the patient's medical and nutritional status. Most physicians tend to use the following format for recording lab values:

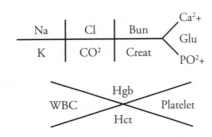

Key:

Na	Sodium	Ca²+	Calcium
K	Potassium	Glu	Glucose
Cl	Chloride	PO²+	Phosphorus
CO²	Carbon oxide	WBC	White blood cells
BUN	Blood urea nitrogen	Hgb	Hemoglobin
Crea	Creatinine	Hct	Hematocrit

See **Table 1–3** for a more detailed description of these items.

REVIEW OF MEDICATIONS

Review of medications and potential food–drug interaction is important in assessing a patient's nutritional status. This section examines the categories of drugs with emphasis on their nutritional implications. The nutritional implications listed are by no means exhaustive, and you should consult food–medication interaction texts for more details; for example, Zaneta M. Pronsky, *Food–Medication Interactions*, 15th ed. (Pronsky, Z. M., 2008).

Because most drugs are metabolized in the liver, patients with a history of liver disease should have liver function tests done regularly.

See **Table 1–4** for detailed explanations of the nutritional implications of classes of drugs.

(text continues on page 54)

Table 1–3 Biochemical Data

Lab Test	Reference Range	Comments
Albumin	3.5–5.0 g/dL	Albumin values should be interpreted with caution because values can be increased with dehydration and steroid use. Values are usually low with edema/ascites, cancer, liver and kidney disease, and malnutrition. Decreases with prolonged hospital stay and immobility. Because of its 21-day half-life, albumin does not give acute changes in nutritional status.
Prealbumin	16–40 mg/dL	Because of its short half-life of about 2 days, prealbumin is more sensitive to acute changes in nutritional status; it is, however, affected by inflammation. Prealbumin level is usually checked whenever a patient is started on enteral/parenteral nutrition.
Blood urea nitrogen (BUN)	8–23 mg/dL	End product of protein metabolism. Increases with dehydration, renal dysfunction, high protein intake, protein catabolism, gastrointestinal hemorrhage, and diabetes. BUN decreases with overhydration, malnutrition, and liver disease.
Calcium	8.5–10.8 mg/dL	50% of calcium is bound to albumin; the rest is ionized calcium. A low calcium level may be caused by poor protein intake. It also decreases with elevated phosphorus and disorders of vitamin D metabolism. Excessive use of intravenous fluids will decrease albumin and thus decrease serum calcium. Calcium increases with cancer and hyperparathyroidism. Carbohydrates increase the intestinal absorption of calcium. For the patient with chronic kidney disease, corrected calcium is equal to $(4.0 - \text{Albumin}) \times 0.8 + \text{Calcium}$.
Creatinine	0.7–1.5 mg/dL	Creatinine increases with kidney disease, dehydration, excessive exercise, starvation, hyperthyroidism, diabetic acidosis, muscular dystrophy, obstruction of the urinary tract, and high protein intake.
Sodium	136–145 mEq/L	Decreased sodium level, or hyponatremia, usually is indicative of fluid overload rather than low serum sodium. It is associated with severe burns, diarrhea, vomiting, excessive IV fluids, diuretics, SIADH, edema, diabetic acidosis, and severe nephritis. Sodium level increases with dehydration, primary aldosteronism, Cushing's disease, and diabetes insipidus.

Lab Test	Reference Range	Comments
Chloride	95–103 mEq/L	Alteration in serum chloride is hardly a primary problem. It is, however, significant in monitoring acid–base balance and water balance. Chloride levels decrease with severe vomiting, diarrhea, ulcerative colitis, severe burns, diabetic acidosis, overhydration, fever, infections, and use of drugs such as diuretics. It is increased with dehydration, anemia, and cardiac decompensation.
Potassium	3.5–5.0 mEq/L	Potassium controls the rate and force of contraction of the heart muscles. Most frequent causes of potassium deficiency/depletion are gastrointestinal loss and IV fluid administration without adequate potassium supplements. Other factors associated with hypokalemia are potassium-depleting diuretics, steroid and estrogen use, malnutrition, renal disease, liver disease with ascites, chronic stress, and fever. Hyperkalemia (increased levels of > 5.5) is frequently caused by renal failure. Cell damage as in burns, accidents, surgery, and chemotherapy causes a release of potassium into the blood, thereby causing hyperkalemia. Other factors include acidosis, internal hemorrhage, uncontrolled DM, and overuse of potassium supplements.
Ammonia (NH^3)	30–70 ug/dL	Ammonia is an end product of protein metabolism and is converted to urea by the liver. Increased ammonia in the blood affects brain function. Increased ammonia levels occur in liver disease, azotemia, severe heart failure, pulmonary disease, and Reye's syndrome. A high-protein diet and vigorous exercise also can cause an increase in ammonia level.
Phosphorus	2.6–4.5 mg/dL	Phosphorus is regulated by the kidneys, and elevated levels are associated with kidney dysfunction and uremia. Other factors associated with hyperphosphatemia (increased phosphorus level) include hypoparathyroidism, excessive intake of vitamin D, hypocalcemia, and Addison's disease. Low phosphorus level is associated with hyperparathyroidism, rickets or osteomalacia, diabetic coma, hyperinsulinism, and overuse of phosphate binders. Whenever phosphorus level is decreased, calcium is increased, and whenever calcium is decreased, phosphorus is increased.

(continues)

Table 1–3 Biochemical Data (continued)

Lab Test	Reference Range	Comments
Hemoglobin (hgb)	F: 12–16 g/dL M: 13.5–17.5 g/dL	Hemoglobin transports oxygen and carbon dioxide. Anemia occurs when hemoglobin, hematocrit, and/or red blood cell count numbers are low. Low hemoglobin levels are associated with cirrhosis of the liver, severe hemorrhage, hyperthyroidism, severe burns, systemic diseases such as Hodgkin's disease, leukemia, and systemic lupus erythematosus. Some HIV medications are associated with anemia. Increased levels of hemoglobin are associated with polycythemia (an increased production of red blood cells), dehydration, COPD, and congestive heart failure.
Hematocrit (hct)	F: 35–45% M: 39–49%	A decreased hematocrit value indicates anemia. Like hemoglobin, low levels are also associated with cirrhosis of the liver, hyperthyroidism, leukemia, severe burns, prosthetic heart valves, and acute massive blood loss. Levels are elevated with polycythemia and severe dehydration.
Red blood cells (RBC)	F: 3.5–5.5 M/mm³ M: 4.3–5.9 M/mm³	Red blood cells are found in the red bone marrow and transport oxygen and carbon dioxide. Anemia results when RBCs are low in conjunction with low hemoglobin (hgb) and hematocrit (hct) levels. The conditions that are associated with low hgb/hct are the same for low RBCs. There is a normal decrease in RBC during pregnancy due to an increase in body fluids. Levels are elevated with polycythemia and severe dehydration.
Ferritin	F: 12–150 ng/mL M: 15–200 ng/mL	Ferritin is the primary storage form of iron in the body. Decreased ferritin value is associated with Iron (Fe) deficiency anemia. Values increase with iron overload, inflammatory diseases, chronic renal failure, malignancy, and hepatitis.
Mean corpuscular hemoglobin (MCH)	26–34 pg/RBC	The MCH is an expression of the average weight of the hemoglobin in the red blood cell. An increase in MCH is associated with macrocytic anemia. Hyperlipidemia will cause a false increase in MCH. A decrease in MCH is associated with microcytic anemia.

Lab Test	Reference Range	Comments
Mean corpuscular hemoglobin concentration (MCHC)	32–37 g/dL	The MCHC is an expression of the average concentration of hemoglobin in the red blood cell. Decreased values are associated with iron deficiency, macrocytic anemia, and thalassemia, an inherited blood disorder characterized by abnormal hemoglobin. Hypochromic anemia is characterized by an MCHC of 30 or less (Fischbach, 2003). An increase in MCHC usually indicates spherocytosis, an inherited disorder of red blood cells where the red cells are smaller, rounder, and more fragile than normal. They tend to get trapped in the spleen, where they break down. MCHC is not increased in pernicious anemia.
Mean corpuscular volume (MCV)	87–103 um³/RBC	The MCV indicates whether the red blood cell appears normocytic, microcytic, or macrocytic, which is used to classify anemias. If the MCV is greater than 103 mm³, the red cells are macrocytic; if they are within normal range, the red blood cells are considered normocytic. Increased MCV values are associated with vitamin B_{12} and folate deficiency.
Total iron binding capacity (Transferrin Test)	240–450 ug/dL 200–400 mg/dL	Transferrin regulates iron absorption and transport in the body. Total iron binding capacity (TIBC) reflects the transferrin content of the blood. An increased TIBC reflects iron-deficiency anemia, whereas a decrease in TIBC reflects iron overload as in chronic inflammatory disease, pernicious anemia, sickle cell anemia, chronic infection, hepatic disease, nephrotic syndrome, cancer, and malnutrition.
Magnesium (Mg)	1.3–2.1 mEq/L	Magnesium deficiency is rare in a normal diet. Mg is important in the absorption of calcium and calcium metabolism. Low levels of Mg occur in the patient with a history of malnutrition, chronic diarrhea, alcoholism, ulcerative colitis, hepatic cirrhosis, hyperthyroidism, and hypoparathyroidism. Increased levels may be seen in dehydration, use of antacids containing Mg such as milk of magnesia, diabetic acidosis, Addison's disease, and hypothyroidism.

(continues)

Table 1–3 Biochemical Data (continued)

Lab Test	Reference Range	Comments
Glycosylated hemoglobin (HgbA1c)	Nondiabetic: 4.0–6.0% Diabetic: < 7.0% A1c Avg Glu 4.0–6.0 60–120 6.1–7.0 121–150 7.1–8.0 151–180 8.1–10.0 181–240 10.1–12.0 241–300 12.1–13.0 301–330	This test provides information on the efficacy of treatment for blood glucose. The more glucose the red blood cell is exposed to, the higher the percentage of glycosylated hemoglobin. Splenectomy decreases life span of red blood cells, so may give a falsely increased level. Hemolysis, on the other hand, gives a falsely decreased level.
Glucose	• 70–110 g/dL Fasting (normal) • 110–125 g/dL Fasting (defined by the American Diabetes Association to be prediabetic) • > 126 g/dL Fasting (on 2 occasions, defined by ADA as diabetes)	Blood glucose is regulated by *glucagon*, which causes an increase in glucose, and *insulin*, which causes a decrease in glucose levels. Increased blood sugar (*hyperglycemia*) usually indicates diabetes but is also associated with other conditions such as acute stress (myocardial infarction, meningitis, and encephalitis), Cushing's disease, hyperthyroidism, pancreatitis, adenoma of the pancreas, brain damage, use of steroids, diuretics, and chronic malnutrition. Low blood sugar (*hypoglycemia*) is associated with overuse of insulin, bacterial sepsis, Islet carcinoma of the pancreas, hepatic necrosis, glycogen storage disease, and hypothyroidism.
High-density lipoprotein (HDL)	Desirable F: > 40 mg/dL M: > 50 mg/dL	HDL is referred to as "good" cholesterol because it is believed that HDL serves as carriers that remove cholesterol from the peripheral tissues and transport it back to the liver for catabolism and excretion. A high level of HDL is an indication of a healthy metabolic system. HDL is increased with exercise. Decreased values are associated with an increased risk for CHD. Cigarette smoking, end-stage liver disease, diabetes, obesity, hyperthyroidism, and increased triglyceride are also associated with decreased HDL values.

Lab Test	Reference Range	Comments
Low-density lipoprotein (LDL)	Desirable: < 130 mg/dL < 100 mg/dL for DM < 70 mg/dL with an occurrence of coronary artery disease (CAD)	Increased LDL levels are caused by a family history of hyperlipidemia, a diet high in cholesterol and saturated fat, nephrotic syndrome, multiple myeloma, diabetes, hepatic disease, and pregnancy. High LDL, referred to as "bad cholesterol," is associated with coronary artery disease.
Triglycerides	< 150 mg/dL	Triglycerides account for about 95% of the fat stored in tissues. Increased triglyceride by itself does not indicate a risk factor for cardiovascular disease (CVD). Levels are increased in pancreatitis, poorly controlled diabetes, myocardial infarction, nephrotic syndrome, liver disease, and hypothyroidism. Levels are decreased with malnutrition, malabsorption, and hyperthyroidism.
Chol/HDL Ratio	**Male** **Female** < 4.2 < 3.9 4.2–7.3 3.9–5.7 7.4–11.5 5.8–9.0 > 11.5 > 9.0	Level of Risk Low average risk Average risk Increased average risk High average risk
Cholesterol, total	Desirable: 120–199 mg/dL	High levels of cholesterol are associated with atherosclerosis, a risk of coronary artery disease. Hypothyroidism, uncontrolled diabetes, nephrotic syndrome, and obesity are conditions associated with high cholesterol. Cholesterol levels are decreased when there is malabsorption, liver disease, hyperthyroidism, anemia, sepsis, stress, use of antibiotics, malnutrition, terminal stages of diseases such as cancer, severe infections, and pernicious anemia.

Note: Please note that reference values vary slightly from one lab to another. ADA = American Diabetes Association; Avg Glu = average glucose; CHD = coronary heart disease; COPD = chronic obstructive pulmonary disease; DM = diabetes mellitus; F = female; M = male; SIADH = syndrome of inappropriate antidiuretic hormone secretion

Table 1–4 Nutrition Implications of Certain Classes of Medications

Medications	Nutritional Implications
Analgesics Examples include MS Contin, Percocet, Nonsteroidal anti-inflammatory drugs (NSAIDs)	Monitor for constipation especially with Oxycontin and Percocet. Take with food to decrease gastrointestinal effect.
Antacids Examples include Maalox, Mylanta, Amphojel	Aluminum-containing antacids should not be used by older persons with bone problems or with Alzheimer's disease. The aluminum may cause their condition to worsen. Take Fe++ separately by 2 hours. Increased fluids are required to prevent constipation.
Antianemic Examples include ferrous sulfate, ferrous gluconate, Epogen, Aranesp	Ferrous sulfate contributes to constipation. Increased fluid is required and a stool softener is usually added to the regimen to alleviate constipation. Ferrous sulfate should be given in conjunction with Epogen for good effect. Frequent iron studies are essential. Monitor for hemachromatosis (iron overload).
Antibiotics Examples include cephlosporins, penicillin, aminoglycosides	The most common side effects of antibiotics are GI distress and diarrhea. Increased intake of fluids and electrolytes is encouraged.
Anticoagulants Examples include Coumadin	Increased risk of GI bleeding evidenced by black tarry stools, bleeding gums, blood in urine/stools, blotches under the skin, shortness of breath, and sudden weakness. Anticoagulants decrease platelets.
Anticonvulsants Examples include Tegretol, phenobarbital, Neurontin, Dilantin, Depakene, Depakote	Drugs such as phenobarbital and Dilantin interfere with intestinal absorption of calcium by increasing vitamin D metabolism in the liver. Long-term use of these drugs may lead to osteomalacia or rickets in children. Tube feeding decreases the bioavailability of Dilantin. Tube feeding should be stopped 2 hours before and after administering the drug.
Antidepressants Examples include Prozac, Zoloft, Luvox Paxil, Celexa, Wellbutrin	May cause dry mouth, blurred vision, constipation, fatigue, loss of appetite, and weight loss.
Antidiarrheals Examples include Kaopectate, Lomotil, Imodium	Diarrhea may increase fluid and electrolyte needs. May cause constipation, dry mouth, nausea, vomiting.

Medications	Nutritional Implications
Antiemetics Examples include Reglan, Compazine, Phenergan	May cause dry mouth, constipation, or diarrhea. May alter insulin requirements in people with diabetes.
Anti-GERD/proton pump inhibitors Examples include, Prevacid, Protonix	Proton pump inhibitors (PPIs) reduce gastric acid production. It is best for patients to take them before meals. PPIs may decrease absorption of iron and vitamin B_{12}.
Antigouts Examples include Zyloprim	Zyloprim is used to treat gouty arthritis, which occurs as a result of too much uric acid in the blood. Alcohol increases uric acid production and therefore should be limited or avoided. Excess amounts of vitamin C increase the risk of kidney stone formation while on Zyloprim. Lots of fluids are encouraged for adequate urine output.
Antihyperlipidemics These include: 1. Statins—for example, Lipitor, Pravachol 2. Fibrates—for example, Lopid, Tricor 3. Niacin—for example, Niacor, Niaspan 4. Resin—for example, cholestyramine (L-cholest, Questran)	Used to improve abnormal lipid values. Side effects include but not are limited to diarrhea, constipation, vomiting, joint and muscle pain, gas, headache, unusual bleeding or bruising, and loss of appetite. Medication is used in combination with a low-fat, low-cholesterol diet.
Antihypertensives/Diuretics Examples include Aldactone, Lasix, calcium channel blockers, ACE inhibitors	Aldactone is potassium sparing, while Lasix is potassium wasting. Potassium levels should be monitored frequently.
Antimanics Examples include lithium	Side effects of lithium include weakness, nausea, fatigue, increased thirst and urination. Consistent sodium intake is required to stabilize the drug level. Extra fluids are required, approximately 2–3 L/day.
Antineoplastics Examples include Thiotepa, Chlorambucil, etoposide phosphate	Common side effects include decrease in the number of blood cells in the bone marrow, nausea, vomiting, constipation, diarrhea, and quite often a change in taste. Loss of appetite and weakness also occur. Increased fluid intake is necessary. Unusual bleeding and/or bruising may occur.

(continues)

Table 1–4 Nutrition Implications of Certain Classes of Medications (continued)

Medications	Nutritional Implications
Antipsychotics Examples include Risperdal, Zyprexa, Seroquel, Haldol	May cause weight gain. Diet and exercise are important to manage weight. Dry mouth, increased salivation, and constipation are also some other side effects.
Antiretrovirals Examples include protease inhibitors (PIs), non-nucleoside reverse transcriptase inhibitors (NNRTIs), and nucleoside reverse transcriptase inhibitors (NRTIs)	Common side effects to antiretroviral therapy include lipodystrophy, insulin resistance, lactic acidosis, hyperlipidemia, osteoporosis/osteopenia, and hepatotoxicity. Loss of appetite, diarrhea, and subsequent weight loss may also occur.
Antirheumatics Examples include methotrexate	Methotrexate is used to treat rheumatoid arthritis and some neoplastic disease. Its side effects include decreased appetite, diarrhea, nausea/vomiting, mouth sores, and possibly unusual bruising/bleeding. It should not be taken with pain medication because this increases the effect of the drug. Alcohol intake with methotrexate can cause very serious liver damage. Methotrexate blocks folic acid synthesis. Folinic acid is used to reduce this side effect associated with use of the drug. Increased fluid intake is encouraged to increase urine output.
Antituberculosis Examples include Rifampin, pyrazinamide (PZA), isoniazid (INH)	May increase glucose in patients taking sulfonylureas for diabetes. Increased uric acid occurs with Rifampin and pyrazinamide. Isoniazid affects vitamin D metabolism, thereby causing a decrease in calcium and phosphorus. High-tyramine foods should be avoided. Isoniazid may also cause liver damage, especially in patients older than 50 years of age.
H¹-Antagonists (antihistamines) Examples include Claritin, Benadryl, Allegra, Zyrtec	Antihistamines are used to relieve allergy symptoms. Side effects may include dry mouth/throat, confusion, headache or tachycardia, blurred vision. Should not be used in combination with Periactin also an antihistamine used to improve appetite.

Medications	Nutritional Implications
Hypnotics/Sedatives Examples include Klonopin, Xanax, Valium, Ativan, BuSpar	May cause bradycardia, heart palpitation, hypotension, nausea/vomiting, dry mouth, constipation, dizziness in coordination, and confusion.
Laxatives Examples include Senna, Dulcolax, Lactulose	Electrolyte imbalance may occur with excessive use. Increased fluid intake is needed with lactulose to prevent constipation. Monitor electrolytes with long-term use.
Muscle Relaxants Examples include Lioresal, Robaxin	May cause epigastric distress. Patients should take these with food to decrease gastrointestinal distress.
Nonsteroidal anti-inflammatory drugs (NSAID) Examples include aspirin, Ecotrin, Bufferin, Motrin	May exacerbate ulcer disease, gastritis, and gastroesophageal reflux disease. Aspirin may cause bleeding, especially in those patients using anticoagulants.
Oral hypoglycemics *Sulfonylureas*—Glucotrol, Glyburide *Biguanide*—Glucophage *Meglitinides*—Prandin *Thiazolidinediones (TZD)*—Actos, Avandia (insulin sensitizers) *Alpha-glucosidase inhibitors*—Precose, Glyset	Glucophage reduces hepatic glucose production. It causes weight loss and an increase in creatinine levels. Patients should avoid alcohol with oral hypoglycemic medication because it can cause a drop in blood sugar. Precose, Glyset decrease the absorption of complex carbohydrates in the upper GI tract, thereby reducing postprandial hyperglycemia. Recent studies indicate that there is a potential risk for developing heart-related conditions with the use of Avandia.
Steroids Examples include systemic steroids such as prednisone, and inhaled steroids	May increase blood sugar in the patient who is predisposed to diabetes. May also cause GI bleeding/perforation. Osteoporosis may occur with long-term use.
Thyroid preparations Examples include Synthroid	May cause weight gain. Iron decreases absorption—patients must take it separately by 4 hours.

Note: GI = gastrointestinal.

SUMMARY

Reviewing the patient's medical chart and taking an in-depth look at the nutritional implications of the disease/medical condition and food–drug interactions and having a clear understanding of the laboratory data provides you with the tools necessary to formulate a proper plan of care for the patient. The chart review also helps you to prepare for the patient interview and educate the patient accordingly.

REVIEW QUESTIONS

1. A 32-year-old woman with below knee amputation (BKA) is admitted to your facility. She weighs 204 pounds and reported her height was 5 ft 9 in. Calculate her adjusted IBW.
2. Patient HS is an 82-year-old woman who is a resident in a nursing home. She does not ambulate, uses a geri-chair, and has a history of constipation. Her height is 62 inches and actual weight is 180 pounds. Patient is fed via G-tube. Formula provides 1200 cal, 54 g protein, and 780 cc water.

Biochemical data: Alb 3.0 BUN 24 Na 134 Ca 7.7 Ammonia 68
Modular: Promod 2 scoops via GT TID
Fluids: 100 cc water flushes administered before and after feeding, 200 cc q shift and 25 cc automatic water flush every hour × 13 hr/day

Patient was noted with a 5% weight gain in 1 month. Evaluate the patient's nutritional status and provide a recommendation for the MD.

REFERENCES

Ayello, E. A., & Cuddington, J. (2004, March). Conquer chronic wounds with wound bed preparation. *Nurse Practitioner: The American Journal of Primary Health Care, 29*(3), 8–25.

Bartlett J. G., & Gallant, J. E. (2005). *Medical management of HIV infection.* Baltimore: Johns Hopkins University Press.

Beckrich, K., & Aronovitch, S. A. (1999). Hospital-acquired pressure ulcers: A comparison of costs in medical vs surgical patients. *Nursing Economics, 17,* 263–271.

Bernard, D. K., & Shaw, M. J. (1993, August). Principles of nutrition therapy for short bowel syndrome. *Nutrition in Clinical Practice, 8,* 153–162.

Bini, L., Fantini, L., Pezzilli, R., Campana, D., Tomassetti, P., Casadei, R., Calculli, L., & Corinaldesi, R. (2007). Medical therapy of malabsorption in patients with head pancreatic resection. *Journal of the Pancreas, 8*(2), 151–155.

Buchman, A. (2004). The medical and surgical management of short bowel syndrome. *Medscape General Medicine, 6*(2), 12.

Burkhead G., Maki, G., AIDS Institute. (2001, March). *Mental health care for people with HIV infection: HIV clinical guidelines for the primary care practitioner.* New York: New York State Department of Health.

Centers for Disease Control and Prevention. (2009). *HIV/AIDS Today.* Retrieved October 1, 2009, from http://www.cdcnpin.org/scripts/hiv/hiv.asp

Centers for Disease Control and Prevention. (2009a). *FAQs for Health Professionals: Hepatitis A.* Retrieved October 1, 2009, from http://www.cdc.gov/hepatitis/HAV/HAVfaq.htm#general

Centers for Disease Control and Prevention. (2009b). *FAQs for Health Professionals: Hepatitis B.* Retrieved October 1, 2009, from http://www.cdc.gov/hepatitis/HBV/HBVfaq.htm#overview

Centers for Disease Control and Prevention. (2008). *HIV Incidence.* Retrieved August 15, 2008, from www.cdc.gov/hiv/topics/surveillance/incidence.htm

Desneves, K. J., Todorovic, B. E., Cassar, A., & Crowe, T. C. (2005, December). *Treatment with supplementary arginine, vitamin C and zinc in patients with pressure ulcers: A randomized controlled trial. Clinical Nutrition, 24*(6),979–987.

DiMaria-Ghalili, R. A. (2008). Nutrition risk factors in older coronary artery bypass graft patients. *Nutrition in Clinical Practice, 23*(5), 494–500.

Duncan, K. D. (2007). Preventing pressure ulcers: the goal is zero. Joint Commission Journal on Quality and Patient Safety, *33*(10), 605–610.

Finelli, L., & Bell, B. P. (2008). *Manual for the surveillance of vaccine-preventable diseases* (4th ed.), chapt 4: Hepatitis B.

Fischbach, F. (2003). *Manual of laboratory and diagnostic tests* (7th ed.) New York: Lippincott, Williams & Wilkins.

Heidt, D.G., Burant, C., & Simeone, D. M. (2007, February). Total pancreatectomy: Indications, operative technique, and postoperative sequelae. *Journal of Gastrointestinal Surgery, 11*(2), 209–216.

Henkel, A. S., & Buchman, A. L. (2006). Nutritional support in patients with chronic liver disease. *Nature Clinical Practice: Gastroenterology and Hepatology, 3*(4), 202–209.

Hojo, K., Bando, Y., Itoh, Y., Taketomo, N., & Ishii, M. (2008, March). Abnormal fecal *Lactobacillus* flora and vitamin B_{12} deficiency in a patient with short bowel syndrome. *Journal of Pediatric Gastroenterology and Nutrition, 46*(3), 342–345.

Joslin Diabetes Center and Joslin Clinic. (2009). *Clinical Guideline for adults with diabetes.* Retrieved October 1, 2009, from http://www.joslin.org/Files/Adult_guidelines_041109_grade_updating.pdf

Klein, C., Stanek, G. S., & Wiles, C. E. (1998). Overfeeding macronutrients to critically ill adults: Metabolic complications. *Journal of American Dietetic Association, 98*, 795–806.

Kopp-Hoolihan, L. (2001). Nutrition and therapeutic effects of probiotics. *Journal of American Dietetic Association, 101,* 229–238, 241.

Lean, M. (2008). Malnutrition in hospitals. *British Medical Journal, 336,* 290.

Mahan, K. L. & Escott-Stump, S. (2008). *Krause's food and nutrition therapy* (12th ed.). St. Louis, MO: Saunders.

Morbidity and Mortality Weekly Report (MMWR). (October 3, 2008). *HIV/AIDS in the United States, 57*(39), 1073–1076.

National Center for Immunization and Respiratory Diseases, Centers for Disease Control and Prevention. (2009, May). *Hepatitis B and hepatitis B vaccine [slideshow].* Retrieved September 15, 2009, from http://www.cdc.gov/vaccines/pubs/pinkbook/downloads/Slides/HepB11.ppt

National Cholesterol Education Program. (2001, May). *Third report of the National Cholesterol Education Program (NCEP) Expert Panel on detection, evaluation, and treatment of high blood cholesterol in adults (Adult Treatment Panel III) executive summary.* Washington, DC: National Heart, Lung, and Blood Institute, National Institutes of Health. NIH Publication No. 01-3670. Retrieved October 1, 2009, from http://www.nhlbi.nih.gov/guidelines/cholesterol/atp_iii.htm

National Institutes of Health, National Institute on Aging. (2005, April). *Aging hearts and arteries: A scientific quest.* NIH Publication No. 05-3738. Bethesda, MD: Office of Communications and Public Liaison.

National Institutes of Health. (2002). *Management of hepatitis C: 2002.* Consensus Conference Statement, June 10–12. Retrieved September 15, 2009, from http://consensus.nih.gov/2002/2002HepatitisC2002116html.htm

National Institute for Health and Clinical Excellence. (February 22, 2006). Nutritional support in adults: Oral nutrition support, enteral, tube feeding and parenteral nutrition. Retrieved October 1, 2009, from http://www.nice.org.uk/guidance/CG32

National Institute of Neurological Disorders and Stroke. (October 19, 2009). Retrieved October 1, 2009, from http://www.ninds.nih.gov/disorders/md/md.htm

Pronsky, Z. M. (1997). *Food–medication interactions* (10th ed.). Birchunville, PA: Food Medication Interactions.

Rich, M. W., Keller, A. J., Schechtman, K. B., Marshall, W. G. Jr., & Kouchoukos, N. T. (1989, March). Increased complications and prolonged hospital stay in elderly cardiac surgical patients with low serum albumin. *American Journal of Cardiology, 63*(11), 714–718.

Russo, C., & Elixhauser, A. (2006). *Hospitalizations related to pressure sores, 2003.* Retrieved October 1, 2009, from http://www.ahrq.gov/news/enews/enews197.htm

Schrader, H., Menge, B. A., Breuer, T. G. K., Ritter, P. R., Uhl, W., & Schmidt, W. E., et al. (2009). Impaired glucose-induced glucagon suppression after partial pancreatectomy. *Journal of Clinical Endocrinology and Metabolism, 94*(8), 2857–2863.

Siitonen, S., Vapaatalo, H., Salminen, S., Gordin, A., Saxelin, M., & Wikberg, R., et al. (1990). Effect of *Lactobacillus* GG yoghurt in prevention of antibiotic diarrhoea. *Annals of Medicine, 22*(1), 57–9.

Spratto, G., & Woods, A. L. (2007). 2008 PDR nurse's drug handbook. Clifton Park, NY: Thomson Delmar Learning.

Teitelbaum, J. E. (2005). Probiotics and the treatment of infectious diarrhea. *Pediatric Infectious Disease Journal, 24*(3), 267–268.

ADDITIONAL RESOURCES

National Cancer Institute: www.cancer.gov

National Institutes of Heath (NIH): www.nih.gov

Centers for Disease Control and Prevention: www.cdc.gov

Doenges, M., Moorhouse, M. F., & Murr, A. (2008). *Nursing Diagnosis Manual: Planning, Individualizing and Documenting Client Care* (2nd ed.). Philadelphia, PA: F. A. Davis Company.

2

The Interview

T he interview is part of the first step in the Nutrition Care Process. It provides additional information that is not found in the chart, and as such, you need to pose open-ended questions and not be judgmental, but be a good listener. Listening carefully shows that you care. The aim is to obtain as much information as possible to conduct a complete and thorough nutrition assessment. Speak clearly and slowly. Questions should be concise and specific without room for ambiguity.

Use the patient's primary language during the interview and make use of the language bank in your facility. If you use a translator for the interview, always introduce yourself and the translator. It is very important that when you use a translator you speak directly to the patient rather than asking the translator to ask the questions. The translator should listen for your cue to translate the questions as they are asked. Avoid body language that may be offensive to the patient.

This chapter covers some very important components of the interview, including obtaining weight history, diet history, bowel movement information, eating patterns, race and diseases, culture and dietary practices, religion and dietary practices, and the use of herbal supplements. With this information, you can conduct a thorough assessment of the patient and provide intervention that meets his or her dietary needs.

OBTAINING DIET HISTORY

Following are sample open-ended questions you can use to obtain information on the patient's diet:

Instead of: Did you have breakfast this morning?

Ask: What did you have for breakfast this morning?

Instead of: How is your appetite?

Ask: How much of your meals do you usually consume? Half or more? Or, How many times during the day do you have something to eat?

Instead of: Do you drink?

Ask: What do you normally drink with your meals? What do you drink between meals?

Instead of: Do you drink water?

Ask: What time of the day do you normally drink water?

Instead of: Do you drink alcohol?

Ask: How many times do you have beer, whiskey, or other alcoholic beverages during a given week, if any?

Instead of: Do you have problem chewing or swallowing?

Ask: Does it hurt when you swallow? Do you find yourself coughing a lot while eating or drinking? Do you have difficulty chewing some foods?

Instead of: How are your bowel movements?

Ask: Do you move your bowels every day, every other day, or every three days?

Follow-up questions might be:

How would you describe your bowel movement—hard, soft, watery, or pebbly? Do you find yourself having to strain to move your bowels?

Instead of: Are you on a special diet?

Ask: What foods were you told to avoid?

Other open-ended questions that are useful in obtaining diet history may include the following:

- Who prepares the food at home?
- Who does the shopping?
- Do you obtain food from any other source such as soup kitchen, food pantry?
- What is a typical breakfast, lunch, dinner, or snack for you?
- What time do you normally have breakfast, lunch, dinner, or a snack?
- How often do you eat outside the home? For example, do you eat at a cafeteria at school/work, fast food, restaurants, homes of friends and family? What do you usually order when you eat out? (Charney & Ainsley, 2009)

OBTAINING WEIGHT HISTORY

Weight history is a sensitive issue, especially for the obese patient. *Never* tell a patient he or she is obese.

Sample questions for obtaining weight history for the obese patient might be the following:

"I noticed that your weight is 276 pounds. Is this your usual weight?"
"Are you comfortable with this weight?"
"Have you gained or lost weight recently?"
"How long have you been at this weight?"
"Have you tried losing weight in the past? If yes, what did you do?"
"Was it effective?"
"Are you interested in losing weight?"

As you interview the patient for weight history, always compare current weight with usual body weight and also determine weight loss or gain over a specific period of time. Provide suitable prompts for the patient to give you the time period.

Sample questions might include these:

"Your current weight is 101 pounds. Have you lost weight recently?"
"How much did you weigh before you started losing weight?"
"How long ago was that—a month ago, three months ago, six months ago, a year or more?"

24-HOUR RECALL

The 24-hour recall is not the most reliable tool for collecting information for a complete assessment because patients quite often tell clinicians what they want to hear. It is not a useful tool for interviewing young children and or older adults because of its reliance on memory (Gibson, 2005).

Accuracy in recalling what they ate in the last 24 hours can be a challenge for many people. Most patients have difficulty determining actual portion sizes. Always have on hand actual portion size examples, such as bowls, cups, spoons, plates, or pictures of these items. Food models are great for portion size demonstrations.

To achieve some level of accuracy with 24-hour recalls, it is best to start with the last meal eaten and work your way back to the first meal of the day. It is important to ask the patient about method of food preparation and about any additives, such as salad dressing, whipped cream, sour cream, and so forth. Answers will enable you to achieve a good estimate of caloric intake. Always ask the patient if this intake is typical of a regular day or whether he or she eats differently on the weekends and when dining out.

FOOD FREQUENCY QUESTIONNAIRE

Food frequency questionnaires (FFQ) are most useful when you assess the nutritional status of a large group of people, as was done in the National Health and Nutritional Examination Survey (NHANES) studies. But they are sometimes used for individual assessments, too. An FFQ asks the participant the number of times he or she eats a particular food over a period of time. FFQs provide you with information on the patient's usual intake and enable you to modify the diet to include choices from all the food groups.

THE RELATIONSHIP BETWEEN RACE/ ETHNICITY AND DISEASES

As you proceed with the interview, it is important to bear in mind that some chronic medical conditions are more prevalent among certain ethnic groups and races. *Race*, as defined by Webster's, is "a distinct group of people who share certain inherited physical characteristics." Some of the most common diseases affecting various ethnic groups are discussed in this section.

Hypertension and diabetes are said to be more prevalent among African Americans than their white counterparts. African Americans, Hispanic Americans, Asian Americans, and Native Americans all have an increased genetic predisposition for **diabetes**. Blindness caused by diabetes and kidney failure rank high among African Americans. The reason for this health disparity could be that patients seek treatment too late in the disease process, receive substandard care from their primary care physician, fail to engage in adequate physical activity; food practices and culture could also be contributors.

Asian Americans have the highest rate of **hepatitis B** in the United States. The rate of prevalence among Chinese Americans is five times higher than that in Caucasian Americans (American Liver Foundation, 2006).

Cystic fibrosis is an inherited disease that affects sodium channels in the body and causes respiratory and digestive problems. It is the most common fatal hereditary disorder affecting Caucasians in the United States. It affects about 1 in 2500 Caucasians and 1 in 25 is a carrier of the defective gene. Risk factors include a family history of cystic fibrosis or unexplained infant death.

Hereditary hemochromatosis (HHC), caused by the body absorbing too much iron, is another common genetic disease affecting Caucasians. One out of every 200 to 400 people is thought to carry a genetic mutation that causes HHC.

Systemic lupus erythematosus (**SLE** or **lupus**), a chronic autoimmune disease that is potentially debilitating and sometimes fatal, is three times more common in African American women than in Caucasian women. It is also more common in women of Hispanic, Asian, and Native American descent than in Caucasians.

Sickle cell anemia is an inherited disease of the red blood cells, which can cause attacks of pain and damage to vital organs and can lead to early death. It is more common among African Americans and Hispanics of Caribbean ancestry. Sickle cell anemia also affects people of Arabian, Greek, Maltese, Italian, Sardinian, Turkish, and Indian ancestry.

Thalassemia is a group of inherited diseases of the blood that causes red blood cell deficiencies. The most severe form, **alpha thalassemia**, results in fetal or newborn death and affects mainly individuals of Southeast Asian, Chinese, and Filipino ancestry.

Tay-Sachs disease is a fatal inherited disease of the central nervous system. Affected babies lack the necessary protein for breaking down certain fatty substances in the brain and nerve cells. These substances build up and gradually destroy brain and nerve cells to the point when the entire central nervous system shuts down, causing the child to go blind, be paralyzed, and die by age 5. Tay-Sachs occurs most frequently in descendants of central and eastern European Jews (Fertility Treatment Center, 2009).

Gaucher's disease is the most frequent hereditary lysosomal deposit storage disorder. It is characterized by a deficiency of the enzyme glucocerebrosidase that leads to an accumulation of substrate in the interior of the macrophage lysosomes. It is a multisystemic disease. In the majority of patients, there is hepatosplenomegaly, anemia, and thrombocytopenia. Skeletal involvement is also important and is frequently the most disabling manifestation (Campo, Calabuig, Aquilar, & Estelles, 2004). This disease is commonly found among Jewish people of eastern European ancestry.

UNDERSTANDING CULTURE AND DIETARY PRACTICES

Culture refers to the perspective, practices, and products of a social group. In conducting an interview with the patient, it is important for you to understand the patient's cultural practices.

In the *Journal of Continuing Education in Nursing,* Cuellar, Cahill, Ford, and Aycock (2003) report that by the year 2080, an estimated 51.1% of the population will be Hispanics, followed by African Americans and Asians.

Obtaining information about the patient's beliefs and cultural practices is as important as reviewing his or her medical condition. Cultural practices can significantly affect medical and nutritional outcomes.

In her article, "Best Culturally Competent Communication Tool," Loreno Drago, (2008) suggests using the following open-ended questions, part of which she refers to as the ETHNIC model:

"What do you think may be the reason you have these symptoms?"
"Do you know anyone else who has this condition, and how is it treated?"
"What kinds of medicines, home remedies, or other treatments have you tried for this illness?"
"Is there anything you eat, drink, or do (or avoid) on a regular basis to stay healthy?"
"Are there any foods you eat to treat this condition?"
"How do you prepare these foods and how often do you eat them?"
"Have you sought advice from alternative/folk healers, friends, or other people who are not doctors?" (Drago, 2008)

Most culturally accepted foods are high in sodium and fat and low in calcium from diary products. There is an increased use of coconut milk and meat consumption in the Hispanic community. Coconut milk is high in saturated fat. Other popular food items include rice and beans, boiled or fried plantains, Spanish cheese, yucca (cassava), and sweet beans, that is, beans with condensed milk.

In Caribbean cultures, natural substances are used for healing, including herbs. Ginger tea, for example, is used for stomach pain, garlic for high blood pressure, and sour orange for respiratory congestion, to name a few. Homemade soups such as cow foot and fish tea are thought to give strength and are common items on the weekly menu. Salads are served mainly on Sundays and hardly during the week. Goat meat, oxtail, and codfish are frequently consumed. Most foods are fried or prepared with a lot of oil.

Prayer is another important component of Caribbean cultures. When sick, people of Caribbean cultures pray to God for help before seeking medical attention. They have a strong belief in faith healing.

Rice is a staple food in Asian cuisine, and foods are usually heavily spiced. There is also an increased consumption of pork among people from the Philippines.

Nutritional Implications and Intervention

Because of the high fat, high sodium content of most culturally accepted foods, it is not uncommon for you to see obesity, hyperlipidemia, hypertension, and diabetes among patients from diverse cultures.

Be cautious when counseling different ethnic groups so as not to make too many drastic changes that will lead to noncompliance. Make an effort to find out the ingredients used in cooking so as to better understand the impact that a particular food has on the patient's nutritional status. Listen carefully to patient's fears and concerns to determine their readiness to change. If a patient is on a restricted diet, changes should be timely and gradual.

RELIGION AND FOOD PRACTICES

Religion is a major influence on the foods most people eat. The role of food in cultural and religious practices is complex and varies among individuals and communities. You must be aware of the religious practices of the patient so as to ensure the patient can comply on some level with a therapeutic diet. Diets provided while patients are confined to a facility should meet the patients' religious mandates.

Buddhism

Some Buddhists include fish in their diet, but most are vegetarians. Most do not eat meat and do abstain from all beef products. The birth, enlightenment, and death of the Buddha are the three most commonly recognized festivals for feasting, resting from work, or fasting. Buddhist monks fast completely on certain days of the moon, and they routinely avoid eating any solid foods after the noon hour.

Hinduism

The cow is sacred to Hindus. Some do eat meat, but not beef. Pork, fowl, ducks, snails, and crabs are also avoided. Most Hindus are strict vegetarians. Although the eating of beef is prohibited, milk, yogurt, and butter are allowed. Many devout Hindus fast on the 18 major Hindu holidays, as well as on numerous personal days, such as birthdays and anniversaries of deaths and marriages. They also fast on Sundays and on days associated with various positions of the moon and planets.

Islam

The term *haram* in the Muslim religion refers to those foods that are prohibited such as pork, alcohol, foods that contain emulsifiers (because emulsifiers may be made from animal fats), tinned vegetables that include emulsifiers, frozen vegetables with sauce, particular margarines, and bread or bread products that contain dried yeast. Gelatine can be made from pig and, because pork is *haram*, products containing gelatine are forbidden. Caffeinated drinks such as coffee and tea are sometimes considered *haram*.

Fasting is practiced regularly on Mondays and Thursdays, and more often for six days during Shawwal (the 10th month of the Islamic year) and for the entire month of Ramadan (the ninth month). Fasting on these occasions includes abstention from all food and drink from sunrise to sunset. The fast is broken in the evening by a meal called the *iftar*, which traditionally includes dates and water or sweet drinks, and is resumed again at sunrise.

Judaism

The term *kosher* refers to the methods of processing foods according to the Jewish laws. Meat and dairy products are never consumed at the same meal; in fact, separate cooking utensils are used during the preparation. Kosher and nonkosher foods cannot come into contact with the same plates. Jewish laws dictate the slaughter and removal of blood from meat before it can be eaten. Animals such as pigs and rabbits and creatures of the sea, such as lobster, shrimp, and clams, are prohibited.

Mormonism

Mormonism promotes abstinence from tobacco, alcohol, coffee, tea, chocolate, and illegal drugs. Products from the land, such as grains, fruits, vegetables, and nuts, are to take the place of meats. Meats, sugar, cheeses, and spices are to be avoided. Reason and self-control in eating are expected in order to stay healthy.

Rastafarianism

People who are devoted to Rastafarianism are completely vegetarians. Some Rastafarians eat fish that are no longer than 12 inches. Pork and shellfish are strictly prohibited. The true Rastas eat only **I-tal** food, which is cooked but served in the rawest form possible, without salts, preservatives, or condiments. *I-tal* food is unique food because it never touches chemicals and is completely natural. Drinking preferences are for anything that is herbal, such as tea. Liquor, milk, coffee, and soft drinks are viewed as unnatural. Marijuana is used during religious observances and is considered to have medicinal properties.

Roman Catholicism

The dietary practices of devout Catholics center around the restriction of meat and fasting behaviors on specified holy days. On designated days, Catholics may abstain from all food, or they may restrict meat and meat products. Water or nonstimulant liquids are usually allowed during the fast.

Seventh-Day Adventists

The Seventh-Day Adventist Church promotes a lacto-ovo vegetarian diet. Pork and shellfish are strictly prohibited. Meat, fish, coffee, tea, and alcohol are avoided (Waibel, 2004).

Nutritional Implications and Intervention

The practice of fasting is almost universal across religious groups, and most religions regard it as a mechanism to discipline followers in a humbling way for spiritual growth. Fasting in the absence of water can lead to dehydration. Some religions emphasize strict adherence to a vegetarian diet (vegan), which puts the growing child and older adults at risk for vitamin B_{12} deficiency. Vitamin B_{12} is found only in animal products and is responsible for the formation of DNA and red blood cell count development. In the absence of animal products, vitamin B_{12} supplementation becomes necessary.

During fasting, people with diabetes may experience a drop in blood glucose. Fasting is not recommended for people with diabetes; however, if a patient insists on fasting, explain the nutritional implications of the fast to him or her and give the option to consume some form of carbohydrate to prevent hypoglycemia. It is advisable for the patient to contact his or her physician prior to the fast for possible adjustment of the diabetes medication or insulin for the duration of the fast.

THE USE OF HERBAL SUPPLEMENTS

In the United States, approximately 38% of adults (about 4 in 10) and approximately 12% of children (about 1 in 9) use some form of complementary and alternative medicine (CAM). The most common types of CAM are herbs, vitamins, chiropractic care, relaxation techniques, spirituality, massage, acupuncture, naturopathy, Chinese medicine, guided imagery, Ayurveda, and chelation. The use of herbal/dietary supplements is the mostly commonly used CAM therapy among adults and is greatest among women and those with higher levels of education and higher incomes.

The sale of dietary supplements today is a $30 billion a year business, and older adults are the main target market. Some dietary supplements interfere with conventional medicines and as such, patients should be advised of the risk of serious complications.

In conducting a thorough nutrition assessment, ask about the use of herbal/dietary supplements. Some patients do not consider this important information or realize that it can be potentially dangerous, so do not volunteer this information. The American Dietetic Association suggests using the following four-step process for evaluating dietary supplement use: Ask, Evaluate, Educate, and Document. **Table 2–1** provides a fuller description of the process.

Table 2–1 Evaluating Dietary Supplement Use

ASK:

- What dietary supplements are you taking? (Type—vitamin, mineral, botanical, amino acid, fiber.)
- What antacids or other over-the-counter medications or food products are being consumed that provide supplemental nutrients, herbals, fiber, etc.?
- Why are you taking the dietary supplement(s)? Include review of patient's diagnosis/symptoms for which they may take supplements (e.g., osteoarthritis, heart disease, high blood pressure, night sweats, loss of memory, fatigue).
- How long have you been taking the dietary supplement(s)?
- What dose? How much? (For each, include chemical form; review and photocopy labels.)
- What frequency? How often? (For each.)
- Sources of supplements—over-the-counter or prescribed, Internet, health care provider, etc.
- Manufacturer
- Is it touted as being preventive or to have treatment effects? What does the label claim? Supplemental brochures/materials?
- Who recommended the supplement—media, physician, nurse, dietetics professional, alternative medicine practitioner, friend, family?

EVALUATE:

- Dietary intake (including intake of fortified food or beverages)
- Health status/health history (include lifestyle habits such as smoking, alcohol, exercise)
- Biochemical profile
- Prescribed and over-the-counter medications
- Clinical response
- Adverse events, symptoms

EDUCATE:

- Scientific evidence of benefit and/or effectiveness
- Potential interaction with foods, nutrients, and/or medications or other dietary supplements
- Appropriate dose, brand, and chemical form; duration of supplementation; appropriate follow-up
- Quality of products, manufacturers, good manufacturing practices (United States Pharmacopoeia, Consumer Labs)
- Mechanism of action of the primary active ingredient
- Duration of use
- How to store the dietary supplement
- Administration instructions: with or without food?, potential food-supplement interactions
- Awareness and reporting of any side effects/adverse events, symptoms
- Recommend concurrent dietary changes
- Remember a supplement should *supplement* the diet

DOCUMENTATION:

- List specific supplements and brand name of each supplement being taken
- Record batch number from bottle in case of an adverse event
- Patient perception, expected level of compliance
- Monitor efficacy and safety including health outcomes and adverse effects
- Medication-supplement or supplement-supplement interactions
- Timeline for follow-up

Source: © 2005 Elsevier, Inc. Practice Paper of the American Dietetic Association: Dietary Supplements Journal of the American Dietetic Association, 15 (Vol. 105, Issue 3), 460–470.

Interactions Between Frequently Used Supplements and Conventional Medicines

Blood thinning agents, such as **warfarin/Coumadin** and **Heparin** are prescribed to prevent occurrence or reoccurrence of heart attack in patients who are at risk for heart disease. However, when these medications are used in combination with some dietary supplements, they can cause prolonged bleeding, which can be fatal if left untreated.

St. John's wort, for example, which is used by many people to treat depression, when taken in combination with warfarin can cause prolonged bleeding and has also been reported to reduce the effects of some antihypertensive medications. St. John's wort may also be responsible for reducing the effectiveness of digoxin, used to treat congestive heart failure.

Feverfew, **ginseng**, **garlic**, **ginkgo biloba**, and **ginger** are also examples of supplements that can cause unusual bleeding or bruising when used in combination with warfarin. Ginkgo biloba has been associated with brain hemorrhage and blood clot. Vitamin E is also known to have blood-thinning effects. Garlic, when used with certain medications to treat HIV/AIDS, may decrease the effectiveness of these medications. One such medication is Saquinavir. Use of garlic caplets lead to a significant decline in plasma concentration of Saquinavir (Piscitelli, Burnstein, Welden, Gallicano, Falloon, 2002).

Omega-3 fatty acids found in fish oils are primarily used to reduce the risk of cardiovascular disease and treat immune disorders, but when used in combination with warfarin can cause unusual bleeding and bruising.

Glucosamine, which is promoted to decrease pain and stiffness in osteoarthritis, may worsen insulin resistance in people with diabetes. This may result in the need to increase doses of diabetes medications or possibly add insulin to the regimen (Shane-McWhorter, 2002).

The Consumer Advisory of the U.S. Food and Drug Administration (FDA) in March 2002 warned that **kava**-containing dietary supplements may be associated with liver-related injuries, including hepatitis, cirrhosis, and liver failure (FDA, 2002). Supplements containing kava are promoted to aid in relaxation (e.g., to relieve stress, anxiety, and tension), sleeplessness, menopausal symptoms, and other uses.

FDA warns consumers to avoid red yeast rice products promoted on the Internet as treatment for high cholesterol. FDA testing revealed that the products contain lovastatin, a cholesterol-lowering drug. It further states that red yeast rice products are a threat to health because the possibility exists that lovastatin can cause severe muscle problems leading to kidney impairment. This risk is greater in patients who take higher doses of lovastatin or who take lovastatin and other medicines that increase the risk of muscle adverse reactions. These medicines include the antidepressant nefazodone, certain antibiotics, drugs used to treat fungal infections and HIV infections, and other cholesterol-lowering medications (FDA, 2007).

Liqiang 4 dietary supplement, promoted as being useful for the control of diabetes, is shown to contain glyburide, a drug that could have serious, life-threatening consequences in some people. The FDA warns that people who have low blood sugar or diabetes can receive dangerously high amounts of glyburide by consuming Liqiang 4 (FDA, 2005).

Dietary/Herbal Treatments and Diabetes Type 2

The National Center for Complementary and Alternative Medicine (2008) reports on the safety and effectiveness of six dietary supplements used to treat diabetes. The supplements are alpha-lipoic acid, chromium, coenzyme 10, garlic, magnesium, and omega-3 fatty acids.

The research findings are as follows:

- *Alpha-lipoic acid (ALA)*: A few studies indicate glucose uptake in muscle, insulin sensitivity, and/or weight loss in patients who take

ALA. ALA may significantly lower blood glucose in patients with diabetes, and therefore close monitoring of blood glucose is necessary. ALA may lower blood levels of iron and may interact with some medications such as antacids and decrease the effectiveness of some anticancer drugs.

- *Chromium*: There is not enough evidence to show that chromium is beneficial in the management of diabetes. Chromium can add to insulin in its effect on blood glucose, which can cause the blood glucose level to drop low. The development of kidney problems can be a serious side effect of chromium supplementation in people with diabetes. Other possible side effects include vomiting, diarrhea, and gastrointestinal bleeding.
- *Coenzyme Q10*: There is not enough scientific evidence to support the effectiveness of Coenzyme Q10 (CoQ10) in treating diabetes. It may interact with other medications such as warfarin and some medications used for high blood pressure treatment and cancer chemotherapy.
- *Garlic*: No evidence-based study supports the benefit of garlic in treating type 2 diabetes.
- *Magnesium*: The relationship between diabetes and magnesium is not fully understood, though low levels of magnesium are commonly found in people with diabetes. Some studies have suggested that low magnesium levels may make glucose control worse in type 2 diabetes, but additional studies are needed to establish whether magnesium supplementation is beneficial in treating diabetes.
- *Omega-3 fatty acids (fish oils)*: Randomized clinical trials have found that omega-3 fatty acids lower triglycerides, but have no significant effect on fasting blood glucose, HbA1c, total cholesterol, or HDL cholesterol. Fish oil in high doses can interact with blood-thinning and hypertensive medications.

Nutritional Implications and Intervention

Certain supplements can boost blood levels of certain drugs to dangerous levels. You must ask patients which herbal supplements they are taking and be nonjudgmental when commenting on these products.

By understanding the side effects of these commonly used herbal/ dietary supplements, you can educate your patients to make informed choices. Encourage patients to discuss their use of supplements with their physician and pharmacist (Shane-McWhorter, 2002).

FOOD ALLERGY AND INTOLERANCE

Food allergy and intolerance are more commonly seen in children but can also be present in adults. Obtaining information on any food allergy, adverse reaction, and/or food intolerance is extremely important, especially in an in-patient setting. Food allergy can be fatal if medical intervention is delayed.

Here are some sample questions to ask the patient to help you determine food allergy or intolerance:

"Are there any foods that make you sick after eating them?"
"What symptoms do you experience after eating these foods?"
"What do you do to relieve these symptoms?"
"What foods do you eat in lieu of the foods to which you are allergic?"

Definitions
- *Adverse food reaction:* Generic term referring to any undesirable reaction following the ingestion of food
- *Food allergy:* An abnormal response to food triggered by the body's immune system (National Institute of Allergy and Infectious Diseases, 2009)
- *Food intolerance:* Result of nonimmunologic mechanism as in lactase deficiency, bacterial food poisoning, and pancreatic insufficiency

Symptoms of food allergy include itching in the throat, difficulty swallowing or breathing, diarrhea, vomiting, nausea, abdominal pain, gastrointestinal bleeding, itching of the skin, flushing, eczema, asthma, and hives (urticaria). In severe cases, anaphylaxis may occur, where, in addition to some or all of the preceding symptoms, there is a sudden drop in blood pressure, tightening of the throat, chest pain, cyanosis, shock, and eventual death if not treated in time. A symptom occurring more than 3 or 4 hours after ingesting food is not food allergy.

Major Food Allergens
- Soy
- Wheat
- Cow's milk
- Egg
- Fish
- Shellfish
- Peanuts and tree nuts

A study reported in the *Journal of the American Dietetic Association* found that children with two or more food allergies were shorter based on height-for-age percentiles than those with one food allergy (Christie, Hine, Parker, & Burks, 2002).

Nutritional Implications and Intervention

Most common food allergens are inconspicuously hidden in foods, but when consumed can have very serious, life-strengthening effects. You must alert patients to these hidden allergens and provide alternate foods that will meet their nutritional needs. The Food Allergy and Anaphylaxis Network is an excellent resource for information on food allergy. See **Figure 2–1** below for foods that may contain food allergens as listed on food labels.

The growing child needs calcium, as do adults and older adults. If a patient presents with allergy to cow's milk, then discuss alternate choices to ensure the person receives adequate intake of calcium. Alternate choices include but are not limited to calcium-fortified rice or soy milk, fortified orange juice, tofu, calcium-fortified bread and cereal, fish eaten with bones in, and green vegetables except spinach. (The calcium in spinach is not bioavailable because of the presence of oxalate, which binds with calcium and makes it unavailable to the body.)

Patients should be advised to always have an EpiPen Auto-Injector or Benadryl (diphenhydramine) in immediate reach at home or when eating out because there is a high probability of cross contact in the preparation of some foods. It is best to avoid processed foods to reduce the risk of cross contact with food allergens.

How to Read a Label for a Milk-Free Diet

All FDA-regulated manufactured food products that contain milk as an ingredient are required by U.S. law to list the word "milk" on the product label.

Avoid foods that contain milk or any of these ingredients:

butter, butter fat, butter oil, butter
  acid, butter ester(s)
buttermilk
casein
casein hydrolysate
caseinates *(in all forms)*
cheese
cottage cheese
cream
curds
custard
diacetyl
ghee
half-and-half
lactalbumin, lactalbumin phosphate
lactoferrin
lactose
lactulose

milk *(in all forms, including con-*
  densed, derivative, dry, evaporated,
  goat's milk and milk from other
  animals, low-fat, malted, milkfat,
  nonfat, powder, protein, skimmed,
  solids, whole)
milk protein hydrolysate
pudding
Recaldent®
rennet casein
sour cream, sour cream solids
sour milk solids
tagatose
whey *(in all forms)*
whey protein hydrolysate
yogurt

Milk is sometimes found in the following:

artificial butter flavor
baked goods
caramel candies
chocolate
lactic acid starter culture and other
  bacterial cultures

luncheon meat, hot dogs, sausages
margarine
nisin
nondairy products
nougat

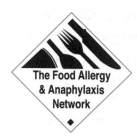

**The Food Allergy
& Anaphylaxis
Network**

11781 Lee Jackson Hwy.
Suite 160
Fairfax, VA 22033-3309
Phone: 703-691-3179
Fax: 703-691-2713
www.foodallergy.org
faan@foodallergy.org

How to Read a Label for a Soy-Free Diet

All FDA-regulated manufactured food products that contain soy as an ingredient are required by U.S. law to list the word "soy" on the product label.

Avoid foods that contain soy or any of these ingredients:

edamame
miso
natto
shoyu
soy *(soy albumin, soy*
  cheese, soy fiber, soy
  flour, soy grits, soy
  ice cream, soy milk,
  soy nuts, soy sprouts,
  soy yogurt)

soya
soybean *(curd, granules)*
soy protein *(concentrate,*
  hydrolyzed, isolate)
soy sauce
tamari
tempeh
textured vegetable protein
  (TVP)
tofu

Soy is sometimes found in the following:

Asian cuisine
vegetable broth

vegetable gum
vegetable starch

Keep the following in mind:

- **The FDA exempts highly refined soybean oil from being labeled as an allergen.** Studies show most allergic individuals can safely eat soy oil that has been highly refined (*not* cold pressed, expeller pressed, or extruded soybean oil).
- Most individuals allergic to soy can safely eat soy lecithin.
- Follow your doctor's advice regarding these ingredients.

How to Read a Label for a Peanut-Free Diet

All FDA-regulated manufactured food products that contain peanut as an ingredient are required by U.S. law to list the word "peanut" on the product label.

Avoid foods that contain peanuts or any of these ingredients:

artificial nuts
beer nuts
cold pressed, expeller pressed, or
  extruded peanut oil
goobers
ground nuts
mixed nuts

monkey nuts
nut pieces
nutmeat
peanut butter
peanut flour
peanut protein hydrolysate

Peanut is sometimes found in the following:

African, Asian *(especially Chinese,*
  Indian, Indonesian, Thai, and
  Vietnamese), and Mexican dishes
baked goods *(e.g., pastries, cookies)*
candy *(including chocolate candy)*
chili

egg rolls
enchilada sauce
marzipan
mole sauce
nougat

Keep the following in mind:

- Mandelonas are peanuts soaked in almond flavoring.
- **The FDA exempts highly refined peanut oil from being labeled as an allergen.** Studies show that most allergic individuals can safely eat peanut oil that has been highly refined (not cold pressed, expeller pressed, or extruded peanut oil). Follow your doctor's advice.

- A study showed that unlike other legumes, there is a strong possibility of cross-reaction between peanuts and lupine.
- Arachis oil is peanut oil.
- Many experts advise patients allergic to peanuts to avoid tree nuts as well.
- Sunflower seeds are often produced on equipment shared with peanuts.

Figure 2–1 How to Identify Food Allergens from Food Labels

How to Read a Label for a Wheat-Free Diet

All FDA-regulated manufactured food products that contain wheat as an ingredient are required by U.S. law to list the word "wheat" on the product label. The law defines any species in the genus Triticum as wheat.

Avoid foods that contain wheat or any of these ingredients:

bread crumbs
bulgur
cereal extract
club wheat
couscous
cracker meal
durum
einkorn
emmer
farina
flour *(all purpose, bread, cake, durum, enriched, graham, high gluten, high protein, instant, pastry, self-rising, soft wheat, steel ground, stone ground, whole wheat)*
hydrolyzed wheat protein
Kamut

matzoh, matzoh meal *(also spelled as matzo, matzah, or matza)*
pasta
seitan
semolina
spelt
sprouted wheat
triticale
vital wheat gluten
wheat *(bran, durum, germ, gluten, grass, malt, sprouts, starch)*
wheat bran hydrolysate
wheat germ oil
wheat grass
wheat protein isolate
whole wheat berries

Wheat is sometimes found in the following:

glucose syrup
soy sauce

starch *(gelatinized starch, modified starch, modified food starch, vegetable starch)*
surimi

How to Read a Label for an Egg-Free Diet

All FDA-regulated manufactured food products that contain egg as an ingredient are required by U.S. law to list the word "egg" on the product label.

Avoid foods that contain eggs or any of these ingredients:

albumin *(also spelled albumen)*
egg *(dried, powdered, solids, white, yolk)*
eggnog
lysozyme

mayonnaise
meringue *(meringue powder)*
ovalbumin
surimi

Egg is sometimes found in the following:

baked goods	Marzipan
egg substitutes	marshmallows
lecithin	nougat
macaroni	pasta

Keep the following in mind:

• Individuals with egg allergy should also avoid eggs from duck, turkey, goose, quail, etc., as these are known to be cross-reactive with chicken egg.

How to Read a Label for a Shellfish-Free Diet

All FDA-regulated manufactured food products that contain a crustacean shellfish as an ingredient are required by U.S. law to list the specific crustacean shellfish on the product label.

Avoid foods that contain shellfish or any of these ingredients:

crab
crawfish *(crayfish, ecrevisse)*
lobster *(langouste, langoustine, scampo, coral, tomalley)*
prawn
shrimp *(crevette)*

Mollusks are not considered major allergens under food labeling laws and may not be fully disclosed on a product label.

Your doctor may advise you to avoid mollusks or these ingredients:

abalone
clams *(cherrystone, littleneck, pismo, quahog)*
cockle *(periwinkle, sea urchin)*
mussels
octopus
oysters
snails *(escargot)*
squid *(calamari)*
Shellfish are sometimes found in the following:
bouillabaisse
cuttlefish ink
fish stock
seafood flavoring *(e.g., crab or clam extract)*
surimi

Keep the following in mind:

• Any food served in a seafood restaurant may contain shellfish protein due to cross-contact.

• For some individuals, a reaction may occur from inhaling cooking vapors or from handling fish or shellfish.

How to Read a Label for a Tree Nut-Free Diet

All FDA-regulated manufactured food products that contain a tree nut as an ingredient are required by U.S. law to list the specific tree nut on the product label.

Avoid foods that contain nuts or any of these ingredients:

almonds
artificial nuts
beechnut
Brazil nuts
butternut
cashews
chestnuts
chinquapin
coconut
filberts/hazelnuts
gianduja *(a chocolate-nut mixture)*
ginkgo nut
hickory nuts
litchi/lichee/lychee nut
macadamia nuts
marzipan/almond paste

Nangai nuts
natural nut extract *(e.g., almond, walnut)*
nut butters *(e.g., cashew butter)*
nut meal
nut paste *(e.g., almond paste)*
nut pieces
nutmeat
pecans
pesto
pili nut
pine nuts *(also referred to as Indian, pignoli, pignolia, pignon, piñon, and pinyon nuts)*
pistachios
praline
shea nut
walnuts

Tree nuts are sometimes found in the following:

black walnut hull extract *(flavoring)*
natural nut extract
nut distillates/alcoholic extracts
nut oils *(e.g., walnut oil, almond oil)*
walnut hull extract *(flavoring)*

Keep the following in mind:

• Mortadella may contain pistachios.

• There is no evidence that coconut oil and shea nut oil/butter are allergenic.

• Many experts advise patients allergic to tree nuts to avoid peanuts as well.

• Talk to your doctor if you find other nuts not listed here.

Source: © 2009 The Food Allergy & Analphylaxis Network, used with permission.

SUMMARY

Interviewing the patient and/or caregiver provides information that you sometimes cannot find in the chart. You can develop trust with the patient during the interview, and the interview provides a foundation on which to build or develop a treatment plan. Phrase questions properly to avoid confusion and ambiguity. Interviews conducted in the patient's primary language produce better results. In some Spanish-speaking groups, similar words have different meanings. Pay special attention to the patient's body language, culture, and religion and be respectful at all times.

REVIEW QUESTIONS

1. Patient SH is a 55-year-old man who came to the emergency department with visible bruising on his left arm. He denies falling or hitting his arm anywhere. Medical history reveals heart attack 8 months ago, at which time the patient was placed on Coumadin. Upon interviewing the patient, he reveals he has been taking omega-3 fatty acids and niacin as recommended by his friends to help with his heart condition. What could be the possible cause for the bruising on his arm?

2. JT is a 13-year-old boy who was rushed to the hospital for anaphylactic shock after eating homemade cookies at his friend's home. He knows he has an allergy to nuts, but his friend's mom said there were no nuts in the cookies. Outline a list of questions that you would use to track the source of the allergen.

REFERENCES

American Dietetic Association. (2005). Practice paper of the American Dietetic Association: Dietary supplements. *Journal of the American Dietetic Association, 105*(3), 460–470.

American Liver Foundation. (2006). *Hepatitis B: What you need to know.* Retrieved October 1, 2009, from www.liverfoundation.org/downloads/alf_download_22.pdf

Campo, L. C., Calabuig, A. J. R., Aquilar J. J., & Alonso, E. (2004). Skeletal, anifestation of Gaucher's disease. *Anales de Medecina Interna, 21*(4), 179–182.

Charney, P., & Malone, A. M. (2009). *ADA pocket guide to nutrition assessment* (2nd ed.). Chicago: American Dietetic Association.

Christie, L., Hine, J. R., Parker, J., & Burks, W. (2002). Food allergies in children affect nutrient intake and growth. *Journal of the American Dietetic Association, 102,* 1648–1651.

Cuellar, N. G., Cahill, B., Ford, J., & Aycock, T. (2003). The development of an educational workshop on complementary and alternative medicine: What every nurse should know. *Journal of Continuing Education in Nursing, 34*(3), 128–134.

Drago, L. (2008). *Best culturally competent communication tool.* Retrieved January 15, 2009, from http://hispanicfoodways.com/professionals_education/

Drago, L. (2004, October). *Effective teaching strategies for dietetic professionals counseling Hispanics with diabetes.* Paper presented at the American Dietetic Association's Food and Nutrition Conference and Expo, Anaheim, CA.

Fertility Treatment Center. (2009). *Preimplantation genetic diagnosis: Breaking the "family curse" of genetic disease.* Retrieved September 16, 2009, from http://www.fertilitytreatmentcenter.com/pgd.htm

Food and Drug Administration. (2002, March 25). Consumer advisory: Kava-containing dietary supplements may be associated with severe liver injury. Retrieved September 15, 2009, from http://www.fda.gov/Food/ResourcesForYou/Consumers/ucm085482.htm

Food and Drug Administration. (2005, July). Liqiang 4 dietary supplement capsules. Retrieved September 15, 2009, from www.fda.gov/Safety/MedWatch/SafetyInformation/SafetyAlertsforHumanMedicalProducts/ucm150476.htm

Food and Drug Administration. (2007, August). FDA warns consumers to avoid red yeast rice products promoted on Internet as treatments for high cholesterol found to contain unauthorized drug. Retrieved September 15, 2009, from http://www.fda.gov/NewsEvents/Newsroom/PressAnnouncements/2007/ucm108962.htm

Gibson, R. (2005). *Principles of nutritional assessment* (2nd ed.). New York: Oxford University Press.

National Institute of Allergy and Infectious Diseases. Retrieved October 1, 2009, from http://www3.niaid.nih.gov/topics/foodAllergy/understanding/whatIsIt.htm

Piscitelli, S. C., Burstein, A. H., Welden, N., Gallicano, K. D., & Falloon, J. (2002). The effect of garlic supplements on the pharmokinetics of Saquinavir. *Clinical Infectious Diseases, 34,* 234–238.

Shane-McWhorter, L. (2002, November 4). Interactions between complementary therapies or nutrition supplements and conventional medications. *Diabetes Spectrum, 15,* 262–266.

Waibel, R. A. (2004). Religion and Dietary Practices. In *Gale Nutrition and Well-Being A to Z.* Retrieved June 1, 2009, from http://www.healthline.com/galecontent/religion-and-dietary-practices

ADDITIONAL RESOURCES

Food Allergy and Anaphylaxis Network: http://www.foodallergy.org
Food and Drug Administration: http://www.fda.gov
National Center for Complementary and Alternative Medicine: http://www.nccam
.nih.gov
Tate, D. M. (2003, September–October). Cultural awareness: Bridging the gap between caregivers and Hispanic patients. *The Journal of Continuing Education in Nursing, 34*(5).

Objective Tools to Collect Information for Assessment

I n addition to chart review and communication with the patient, you can use certain objective tools to collect information. These tools are helpful because they eliminate bias and some degree of subjectivity. This information forms a part of step 1 in the Nutrition Care Process. However, because these tools are handled by individuals the likelihood of human error is possible; use them, therefore, in combination with a thorough nutrition assessment of the patient.

DIRECT OBSERVATION STUDY

Direct observation studies are usually conducted in an in-patient setting and are considered an objective tool for assessing food intake. Here, you observe the patient during mealtime to determine actual intake, refusal of meals, food preferences, difficulty chewing/swallowing, repeated coughing between sips of fluids, positioning, use of utensils, food spillage, and need for adaptive feeding equipment. You might need more than one meal to get a true picture of the patient's oral intake.

Once the observation study is completed, you must document the findings and provide intervention to address need(s). If you observe a patient coughing between sips of fluids, there is a strong possibility that the patient has some swallowing difficulty and should be referred to a speech-language pathologist for further evaluation. Record oral intake in terms of percentage consumed. See the guidelines given in **Figure 3–1**.

Consult an occupational therapist whenever you observe food spillage with regular utensils because the patient could benefit from adaptive feeding equipment to allow for maximum meal intake. Inadequate intake because of food spillage can result in weight loss.

CALORIE COUNT STUDY

The physician in collaboration with the nurse or dietitian may order a calorie count study. Calorie count studies are used to justify the need for nutrition support in the case of patients with poor oral intake and those who have difficulty meeting their nutritional needs. They are also used to initiate the weaning process for the patients who are tube fed and to determine actual caloric intake in patients who are reportedly eating well but still losing weight.

Calorie counts are usually conducted over a 3-day period, but can last longer. A good calorie count study should include the following features:

- The actual oral intake in terms of portions for each food item consumed including snacks, supplements, nourishment, and drinks
- The length of the study
- The calories, carbohydrates, and protein consumed from each food item
- The total calories, carbohydrates, and protein consumed for the day
- The average daily consumption of calories, carbohydrates, and protein
- A comparison between actual intake and daily requirements for calories, carbohydrates, and protein expressed in percentages
- A recommendation for further intervention to address deficiency, if any, based on the outcome of the calorie count study

Give priority to calorie count studies because physicians depend on this information for further evaluation of the patient's medical and nutritional status.

Example: Patient HP is a 35-year-old man who was admitted to the hospital with pneumonia and wasting syndrome secondary to AIDS. He

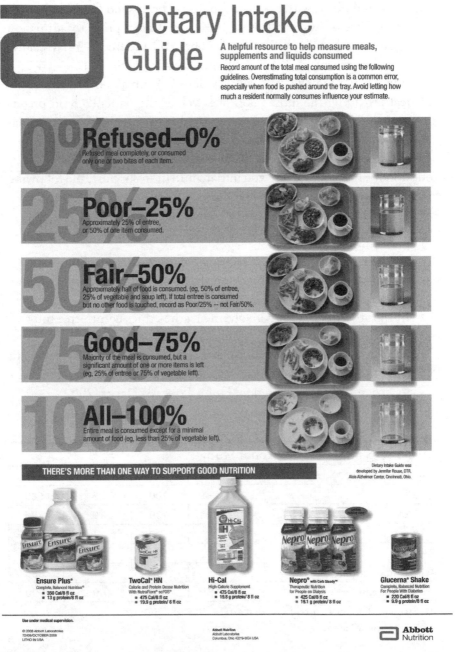

Figure 3–1 Percent Consumed Chart

Source: © 2008 Abbott Laboratories. Used with permission.

is lethargic and noted with poor oral intake on both solid foods and nutritional supplement. Weight loss of 10% in 30 days prior to admission (PTA). Serum albumin is 2.2 mg/dL. The MD ordered a 3-day calorie count for this patient, and the results are listed in **Table 3–1**.

Besides nutrient intake, you can also identify from a calorie count study the meal providing the most calories as well as the patient's food preferences and eating pattern, which can be useful in making recommendations for nutritional intervention.

In the preceding example, the patient is definitely a candidate for nutrition support; however, before you initiate nutrition support, the following criteria must be met:

- The patient with decision-making capacity must consent to the procedure.
- If a patient does not have decision-making capacity, a family member or surrogate must act on that patient's behalf and request the procedure.
- In the absence of family involvement, the ethics committee must meet to approve of the procedure.
- The opinion of the attending physician is that the patient will benefit from the procedure and there is reasonable hope he or she will return to a cognitive state. (Langdon, Hunt, Pope, & Hacks, 2002)

Table 3–1 Sample Calorie Count Study

Day	CHO (g)	Protein (g)	Calories
3/16/09	100	22	680
3/17/09	130	19	775
3/18/09	90	21	600
Total	**320**	**62**	**2055**
Average daily intake	**106**	**21**	**685**
Daily requirements	**275**	**100**	**2000**

Assessment: Patient's current intake meets: < 38% of CHO needs

< 21% of protein needs

< 34% caloric needs

Recommendation: This patient could benefit from alternate feeding to meet nutritional needs because current intake meets < 40 % of daily requirements.

Note: CHO = carbohydrate.

BODY MASS INDEX

Body mass index (BMI) is an objective tool that is used to measure the relationship between a person's height and weight to determine health risks. Being overweight is related to the development of certain diseases such as heart disease and some cancers. Other obesity-related conditions include hypertension, osteoarthritis, sleep apnea and respiratory problems, stroke, gallbladder disease, and dyslipidemia.

BMI values increase with age, so a BMI between 18.5 and 24.9 may be too restrictive for older adults. BMI of 27 is acceptable for adults older than 65 years of age.

Use the guidelines in **Table 3-2** to assess BMI and its implications in adult men and women. Use the following equation to calculate BMI:

$$BMI = \frac{\text{Weight (in kilograms)}}{\text{Height (in meters)}^2}$$

BMI does not differentiate between muscle mass and fat mass, so should be used cautiously when classifying fatness in athletes and nonathletes. Muscles are more dense than fat is. Because of a larger muscle mass among male and female athletes, BMI incorrectly classifies normally fat athletes as overweight (Ode, Pivarnik, Reeves, & Knous, 2007).

Table 3-2 Interpreting Body Mass Index

BMI	Implications/ Interpretation	Health Risks
< 18.5	Underweight	May be associated with health problems, for example, osteoporosis
18.5–24.9	Normal weight	Minimal health risk
25.0–29.9	Overweight	Low to moderate risk. May be associated with health problems in some people
30.0–34.9	Obesity class I	High health risk
35.0–39.9	Obesity class II	Very high health risk
> 40.0	Obesity class III	Very high health risk

Source: Adapted from Clinical Guidelines on the Identification, Evaluation, and Treatment of Overweight and Obesity in Adults: The Evidence Report; 98-4083; 1998. National Heart, Lung, and Blood Institute, National Institutes of Health.

Use BMI values in conjunction with laboratory values, waist circumference, body fat percentage, and lifestyle to determine a patient's actual health risk. Smoking, low high-density lipoproteins (HDL), high low-density lipoproteins (LDL), high cholesterol, and sedentary lifestyle are major risk factors for cardiovascular disease and other serious health problems.

WAIST CIRCUMFERENCE AND WAIST-TO-HIP RATIO

Waist-to-hip ratio is used to measure the distribution of adipose tissue. It differentiates between android obesity (apple shape) where there is an accumulation of fat in the abdominal area, and gynoid obesity (pear shape) where fat is concentrated in the hip and thighs. A waist-to-hip ratio of 1.0 or greater in men, and 0.8 or greater in women, is a risk factor for obesity-related diseases.

Compared with waist-hip ratio, waist circumference has been shown to be a better marker of visceral fat and correlates more strongly with cardiovascular disease risk factors. Waist-to-hip ratio has also been shown to be a good predictor of increased risk of diabetes and CHD. Peripheral fat accumulation in the hips and thighs, for a given amount of abdominal fat, may be associated with a more favorable metabolic profile (Parker, Pereira, Stevens, Folsom, 2009).

A woman with a waist size > 35 inches and a man with a waist size > 40 inches are considered at risk for serious health problems such as heart disease, diabetes, high blood pressure, high cholesterol, sleep apnea, and asthma (National Cholesterol Education Program, 2001).

BODY FAT PERCENTAGE

Body fat percentage refers to the amount of body fat mass compared to total body weight. The body consists of fat mass, bones, connective tissue, blood, muscles, and water. The main stores of fat are subcutaneous and intra-abdominal, and considerable amounts of fat can also reside within muscles, particularly in older adults. After age 50, muscle mass is, to varying degrees, replaced by fat, much of it within the abdomen (Willett, 1999).

Various methods are used to determine body fat percentage. These include but are not limited to the following:

- **Skin fold thickness.** A caliper is used to measure a pinch of skin at various sites on the body to determine subcutaneous fat.
- **Bioelectrical impedance analysis** (BIA). Electrodes are attached to the right hand, wrist, ankle, and foot of the patient and pass a small electrical current through the body. BIA measures the impedance or resistance to the signal as it travels through the water that is found in muscle and fat. Lean tissue has a higher electrical conductivity and lower impedance than fatty tissue does.

Body fat percentage varies among ethnic groups. Gallagher et al. (2000) conducted a study to examine a potential new approach for developing percentage body fat ranges. The approach linked healthy body mass index with predicted percentage body fat. Among African Americans, whites, and Asians, the study found that Asians were shorter than their white and African American counterparts. BMI was lowest in Asian men and women and highest in African American women. Asians also had a significantly higher percentage body fat for any given BMI than did the other two ethnic groups. **Table 3–3** shows the predicted body fat ranges for whites and African Americans, and **Table 3–4** shows the predicted ranges for Asians.

Table 3–3 Predicted Percentage Body Fat Ranges by Sex for African Americans and Whites

Sex and BMI	20–39 Years Old (%)	40–59 Years Old (%)	60–70 Years Old (%)
Women			
BMI < 18.5	21	23	24
BMI ≥ 25	33	34	36
BMI ≥ 30	39	40	42
Men			
BMI < 18.5	8	11	13
BMI ≥ 25	20	22	25
BMI ≥ 30	25	28	30

Source: Gallagher et al., *American Journal of Clinical Nutrition*, Vol 72, Sept., 2000.

Table 3–4 Predicted Percentage Body Fat Ranges by Sex for Asians

Sex and BMI	20–39 Years Old (%)	40–59 Years Old (%)	60–70 Years Old (%)
Women			
BMI < 18.5	25	25	25
BMI ≥ 25	35	35	36
BMI ≥ 30	40	41	41
Men			
BMI < 18.5	13	13	14
BMI ≥ 25	23	24	24
BMI ≥ 30	28	29	29

Source: Gallagher et al., *American Journal of Clinical Nutrition,* Vol 72, Sept., 2000.

INDIRECT CALORIMETRY

"Indirect calorimetry is still widely used to measure resting energy expenditure in patients admitted to the Intensive Care Unit. Indirect calorimetry remains the gold standard in measuring energy expenditure in the clinical setting. It offers a scientifically-based approach to customize a patient's energy needs and nutrient delivery to maximize the benefits of nutrition therapy." (Haugen, Chan, & Li, 2007)

Indirect calorimetry measures energy expenditure. Energy expenditure is quantified under specific conditions (usually resting) by measuring respiratory gases (oxygen consumed and carbon dioxide produced). Here is the equation to calculate energy expenditures:

$$\text{Energy expenditure (Kcal/d)} = [(VO^2 \times 3.941) + (VCO^2 \times 1.11)] \times 1440$$

Respiratory quotient (RQ) reflects substrate use and is defined as the ratio between carbon dioxide production (VCO^2) and oxygen consumption (VO^2). The complete oxidation of glucose in a given system yields an RQ value of 1.0. The higher the RQ, the more carbon dioxide is produced and the greater the demand on the respiratory system. **Table 3–5** gives the respiratory quotient for the three main biological substrates: glucose, fat, and protein.

Resting condition, where there is a minimum of 5 hours of fasting, no physical activity, and abstinence from nicotine, caffeine, and other stimulants is ideal for the measurement of energy expenditure.

Table 3–5 Respiratory Quotient for Biological Substrates

Substrate	Respiratory Quotient
Glucose	1.00
Fat	0.69
Protein	0.81

Both underfeeding and overfeeding critically ill patients can have serious consequences and negatively affect recovery and healing. Overfeeding can result in poor glycemic control, increased risk of infectious complications, delayed weaning from mechanical ventilation, or even death. With indirect calorimetry, you can tailor calories to meet the energy needs of the patient. Quite often caloric requirements are overestimated, especially in the cases of obese patients, thereby increasing the risk of overfeeding.

Consider using indirect calorimetry for patients who are severely malnourished, HIV positive with wasting syndrome and opportunistic infections, and who have been receiving nutrition support, but fail to show clinical responses.

Measuring energy expenditure has been found to be useful in providing nutrition support for the bariatric patient. The risk of developing malnutrition is high in the bariatric patient. Malabsorption is also common, and it is not certain how many calories are actually absorbed. Indirect calorimetry, therefore, provides a more accurate and patient-specific assessment of how many calories the body uses at rest (resting energy expenditure, REE). (Haugen et al., 2007).

NITROGEN BALANCE

The most common clinical method for assessing a patient's protein requirement is determination of nitrogen balance (nitrogen intake minus nitrogen excretion), in which intake represents the patient's nutritional nitrogen and excretion is traditionally the sum of measured urinary nitrogen plus an estimate of cutaneous and gastrointestinal losses. Nitrogen balance calculations, and their improvement over time in response to nutritional therapy, are the nutritional variable most consistently associated with improved patient outcome during critical illness. Achievement of a positive nitrogen balance is widely considered to be the primary goal of nutritional support (Cheatham, Safcsak, Brzezinski, & Lube, 2007).

Nitrogen balance is used to determine anabolism or catabolism. It is calculated from 24-hour urine collection analyzed for urea urinary nitrogen (UUN).

To achieve an accurate nitrogen balance, protein intake must be accurate. If there is decreased urine output, this could affect the result.

The formula to calculate nitrogen balance is as follows:

$$\text{Nitrogen balance} = \frac{\text{Protein (g) intake} - (\text{UUN} + 4)}{6.25}$$

Here is how to interpret the values:

1. A negative balance indicates the patient is in a catabolic state; the goal, therefore, is to achieve two to four positive balances. Adequate nutritional support may be needed to achieve this goal.
2. A positive balance indicates increased lean body mass.
3. A healthy person has a 0 balance.

BONE MINERAL DENSITY TEST

Bone mineral density tests are used to determine a patient's risk of osteoporosis, which occurs as a result of decreased bone mass. It is estimated that 1.24 million osteoporosis-related fractures occur in women each year. The bone mineral density test, though not commonly administered in an acute care setting, remains a good marker for determining risk of fracture. Bone mass decreases with age, especially in women after age 50 or at the time of menopause. Approximately two thirds of osteoporosis-related vertebral fractures are undiagnosed.

Risk factors for osteoporosis includes the following:

- Age, mainly postmenopausal women
- Inadequate calcium and vitamin D intake
- Low body weight
- Cigarette and alcohol use
- Ethnicity and family history
- Inactivity
- Medications—antidepressants, steroids, heparin, antacids containing aluminium, Dilantin (phenytoin) used for seizure disorder, methotrexate, Lasix (furosemide), and thiazide diuretics

- Chronic medical conditions—kidney disease, hyperthyroidism, diabetes, chronic diarrhea, and hemiplegia

A new report issued by the International Osteoporosis Foundation (IOF) and published in the scientific journal *Osteoporosis International* shows that populations across the globe are suffering from the impact of low levels of vitamin D. Suboptimal levels of vitamin D may lead to increased risk of osteoporosis and hip fracture (Mithal et al., 2009).

According to the 2004 report of the Surgeon General on bone health and osteoporosis, half of all women older than age 50 will have an osteoporosis-related fracture in their remaining lifetime (Office of the Surgeon General, 2004).

Though not as common as in women, osteoporosis also affects men. You must assess for the risk factors of osteoporosis when conducting an initial assessment in both men and women. Following are criteria for assessing for osteoporosis:

World Health Organization Diagnostic Criteria for Osteoporosis
- Normal: t score > 1.0
- Osteopenia: t score −1.0 to −2.5
- Osteoporosis: t score less < −2.5

SUMMARY

The use of objective tools in assessing the patient provides additional information you need for a thorough assessment of the patient's nutritional status. This information helps you develop treatment plan and goals to meet nutritional needs. It is, however, important that you understand the limitation of these tools because certain factors, including human error, can alter results. For patients who are overweight, a 5–10% reduction in weight can significantly improve health outcomes.

REVIEW QUESTIONS

1. A morbidly obese patient was intubated in the ICU following a heart attack. You have been asked to assess the patient's caloric needs. Which assessment tool would be most useful in determining this patient's actual caloric needs?

2. Hector is 5 ft 7 in. tall and weighs 200 pounds. Calculate his body mass index. What health risks are associated with his BMI?

REFERENCES

Cheatham M. L., Safcsak, K., Brzezinski, S. J., & Lube, M. W. (2007, January). Nitrogen balance, protein loss, and the open abdomen. *Critical Care Medicine,* 35, 127–131.

Gallagher, D., Heymsfield, S. B., Heo, M., Jebb, S. A., Murgatroyd, P. R., & Sakamott, Y. (2000). Healthy percentage body fat ranges: An approach for developing guidelines on body mass index. *American Journal of Clinical Nutrition, 72,* 694–701.

Haugen, H. A., Chan, L.-N., & Li, F. (2007, August). Indirect calorimetry: A practical guide for clinicians. *Nutrition in Clinical Practice, 22, 377–387.*

Langdon, D. S., Hunt, A., Pope J., & Hackes, B. (2002, June). *Nutrition support at the end of life: Opinions of Louisiana dietitians. Journal of the American Dietetic Association, 102*(6), 837–840.

Mahan, L. K., & Escot-Stump, S. (2008). *Krause's food and nutrition therapy* (12th ed.). St. Louis, MO: Saunders.

Mithal, A., Wahl, D.A., Bonjour, J.-P., et al. (in press). Global vitamin D status and determinants of hypovitaminosis D. *Osteoporosis International.*

National Cholesterol Education Program. (2001, May). *Third report of the National Cholesterol Education Program (NCEP) Expert Panel on detection, evaluation, and treatment of high blood cholesterol in adults (Adult Treatment Panel III) executive summary.* Washington, DC: National Heart, Lung, and Blood Institute, National Institutes of Health. NIH Publication No. 01-3670.

Ode, J. J., Pivarnik, J., Reeves, M., & Knous J. (2007, March). Body mass index as a predictor of percent fat in college athletes and nonathletes. *Medicine and Science in Sports and Exercise, 39*(3), 403–409.

Office of the Surgeon General. (2004). *Bone health and osteoporosis: A report of the Surgeon General.* Rockville, MD: U.S. Department of Health and Human Services, Public Health Service.

Parker, E. D., Pereira, M. A., Stevens, J., & Folsom, A. R. (2009, April 1). Association of hip circumference with incident diabetes and coronary heart disease: The atherosclerosis risk in communities study. *American Journal of Epidemiology, 169,* 837–847.

Willet, W. C., Dietz, W. H., & Colditz, G. A. (1999, August 5). Guidelines for healthy weight. *New England Journal of Medicine, 341,* 427–434.

WHO Scientific Group on the Assessment of Osteoporosis at Primary Healthcare Level. (2004, May 5–7). Summary meeting report. Brussels, Belgium.

WHO Study Group. (1994). *Assessment of fracture risk and its application to screening for postmenopausal osteoporosis.* (WHO Technical Report Series No. 843). Geneva, Switzerland: World Health Organization.

Assessment During Pregnancy and Lactation

T his chapter looks at the nutritional needs of the mother and unborn child as well as the complications associated with pregnancy. It will also consider nutritional care for the lactating mother.

DIETARY ASSESSMENT OF THE PREGNANT WOMAN

The mother's dietary intake prior to and during pregnancy is important and has significant bearing on the outcome of the pregnancy. Conditions associated with poor nutrition during pregnancy include low-birthweight babies (< 2500 g), neural tube defect, and iron-deficiency anemia, which can lead to developmental delays.

It is also important to ascertain the social and psychological history of the mother prior to pregnancy. Use of recreational drugs and alcohol can have deleterious effects on the fetus, resulting in retarded growth. Mothers who are depressed do not usually eat well and they tend to delay prenatal care. Details about drug use and depression are addressed later in this chapter.

The dietary assessment form in **Figure 4–1** was developed by the Connecticut Women, Infants, and Children (WIC) Program.

Diet Assessment—Pregnant Women

1. Before this pregnancy, how many times were you pregnant? _____	8. Are you interested in breastfeeding this baby? ( ) Not sure ( ) Yes ( ) No
2. When was your last child born? _____	9. In this pregnancy, how far along were you when you had your first prenatal exam? (circle the month) Month 1 2 3 4 5 6 7 8 9
3. How many children have you given birth to? _____ ( ) miscarriage > 2 ( ) fetal loss > 20 weeks ( ) neonatal loss < 28 days	10. Before this pregnancy began, how much did you weigh? _____ pounds _____ kg
4. Have you ever had a baby who weighed less than 5 pounds, 8 oz? ( ) No ( ) Yes	11. When is your baby due? MM/DD _____
5. Have you ever had a premature baby (less than 38 weeks)? ( ) No ( ) Yes	**In the three months before you got pregnant:** 12. How much did you smoke? _____ cigarettes a day ( ) not a cigarette smoker ( ) smoke marijuana ( ) use other drugs ( ) smoke other drugs ( ) do not use drugs
6. When did your last pregnancy end? _____	13. How many days per week did you drink alcohol, beer, wine, or wine coolers? _____ days a week ( ) weekends ( ) occasionally ( ) not at all
7. Have you ever breastfed? ( ) No ( ) Yes For how long? _____ Why did you stop? _____	14. How many alcoholic drinks did you have a day? _____

Figure 4–1 Connecticut WIC Program

15. **Now that you are pregnant:** How much do you smoke: _____ cigarettes a day ( ) smoke marijuana ( ) use other drugs ( ) not a cigarette smoker ( ) smoke other drugs ( ) do not use drugs	22. Do you eat or drink the following foods every day? Cereal, bread, or rice ( ) No ( ) Yes Milk, cheese, or yogurt ( ) No ( ) Yes Meat/eggs/beans/ peanut butter ( ) No ( ) yes Fruit or fruit juice ( ) No ( ) Yes Vegetables ( ) No ( ) Yes
16. Has there been a change in the amount you smoke? ( ) no change ( ) stopped completely ( ) increase ( ) decrease ( ) tried to stop but failed ( ) not a smoker	23. Do you have ( ) nausea? ( ) vomiting? ( ) heartburn? ( ) constipation? ( ) problems drinking milk? ( ) allergies? ( ) other_____
17. Does anyone smoke in your home? ( ) No ( ) Yes	24. Do you have cravings for ( ) cigarette ashes? ( ) laundry starch? ( ) ice chips? ( ) corn starch? ( ) other?_____
18. How many days a week do you drink alcohol, beer, wine, or wine coolers? _____ days a week _____ weekends _____ occasionally _____ not at all	25. Would you like to talk about ( ) breastfeeding? ( ) wise food choices? ( ) healthy weight gain? ( ) other
19. How many alcoholic drinks do you have a day? _____	26. What else would you like to share with us? _____ _____
20. Do you take medication? ( ) No ( ) Yes If yes, what kind?_____ Other drugs? ( ) No ( ) Yes Vitamins? ( ) No ( ) Yes Iron/minerals? ( ) No ( ) Yes	
21. Do you use herbal teas? ( ) No ( ) Yes If yes, what kind? _____ Home remedies? ( ) No ( ) Yes_____	OFFICE USE: _____ Nutrition Staff Initials or Signature

Source: Courtesy of Connecticut WIC Program.

NUTRITIONAL NEEDS OF THE PREGNANT WOMAN

Calories

By using the 24-hour food recall, food frequency questionnaire, dietary assessment, and weight record with pregnant women, you can determine adequate caloric intake to meet the demands of pregnancy and development of the fetus. Nausea and vomiting during pregnancy can deprive both mother and fetus of important nutrients. Extreme exercise can decrease weight gain and subsequently affect the growth of the fetus.

Calorie intake for the first trimester is the same as for the nonpregnant woman and is usually calculated as 25–30 cal/kg body weight. Ideal body weight is used in this calculation for the obese woman. During the second and third trimesters, the pregnant woman needs an additional 350–400 cal/day. Although a weight record is helpful in determining adequacy of caloric intake, the presence of edema can cause a shift in weight, which makes weight a less accurate measure of intake.

Protein

Protein requirements increase with pregnancy because of maternal tissue growth as well as rapid fetal tissue growth. High biological value protein is recommended; however, for those women who follow a vegan diet, meals should be properly planned to meet protein needs. Fortified soy, rice, or almond milk in addition to legumes, nuts, and meat analogs are good sources of protein. The U.S. Department of Agriculture (2002) Dietary Reference Intakes (DRIs) suggest 71 g of protein per day for pregnant and lactating women.

Dietary Fiber

With the use of iron tablets and decreased activity, there is an increased risk for pregnant women to become constipated. Diet should provide 25–30 g of fiber daily. As fiber is increased, fluids should also be increased.

Vitamins and Minerals

Whereas most prenatal supplements contain vitamins and minerals, the diet should be rich in iron; folic acid; calcium; fat-soluble vitamins A, D,

E, and K; and the B vitamins as well as vitamin C. Folic acid deficiency has been associated with neural tube defect. Sources of folic acid include peas, beans, dark green leafy vegetables, broccoli, and fortified cereals.

There is a demand for iron during pregnancy and this demand cannot be met by diet only because most women have low iron stores even before pregnancy. Iron supplementation is usually given and should be taken 1–2 hours apart from calcium supplements. During the first two trimesters of pregnancy, iron-deficiency anemia increases the risk for preterm labor, low-birthweight babies, and infant mortality and predicts iron deficiency in infants after 4 months of age (Gautam, Saha, Sekhri, Saha, 2008).

Calcium is needed for the skeletal development of the fetus. Recommended intake is 1000 mg/day for pregnant women 19–50 years of age. Women under 19 should be consuming 1300 mg/day.

Vitamin D intake is important for the absorption of calcium. Low levels of vitamin D during pregnancy are found to be associated with reduced bone mineral accrual in childhood (Javaid et al., 2006). Vitamin D deficiency is considered a risk factor for preeclampsia, a complication of pregnancy characterized by high blood pressure and proteinuria. With limited exposure to the sun and reduced intake of vitamin D–enriched foods, women entering into pregnancy present already with low vitamin D levels. Supplementation is usually required to reduce nutritional risks associated with vitamin D deficiency.

Fluids

Adequate fluid intake is necessary during pregnancy to reduce the risk of constipation and urinary tract infection. Eight to 10 cups of fluids, preferably water, are recommended.

Omega-3 Fatty Acids

Docosahexaenoic acid (DHA) and arachidonic acid (AA) are essential for the development of the central nervous system in mammals. A study conducted by the American Academy of Pediatrics indicates that maternal supplementation with very-long-chain n-3 polyunsaturated fatty acids during pregnancy and lactation improves the intelligence of children at 4 years of age (Hellend, Smith, Saarem, Saugstad, & Drevon, 2003).

The main source of DHA is fatty fish. Omega-3 fatty acids can also be obtained from flaxseed. It is recommended that pregnant women consume two to three fish meals per week. The Food and Drug Administration, however, cautions women of child-bearing age against eating certain fish because of their exposure to mercury and polychlorinated biphenyl (PCB), which can pose harm to the fetus. Shark, swordfish, king mackerel, and tilefish contain high levels of mercury and should be avoided. Shrimp, canned light tuna, salmon, pollock, and catfish are low in mercury and are considered safe to eat. The U.S. Environmental Protection Agency suggests tuna steak be eaten only once per week because of its reported higher levels of mercury. Fish sticks and fast-food fish sandwiches are commonly made from fish that is low in mercury (U.S. Environmental Protection Agency, 2004).

WEIGHT GAIN DURING PREGNANCY

Weight gain during pregnancy is a good predictor of fetal outcome. Weight gain is a combination of increased weight of the breasts, blood, uterus, amniotic fluid, placenta, fluid, maternal fat, and fetus.

Inadequate weight gain can result in babies with low birthweight (< 2500 g) and early labor. The rate of weight gain during pregnancy depends on the woman's weight prior to pregnancy. (See **Table 4–1** for recommendations.) A prospective cohort study found that women with a body mass index of < 19.8 were at higher risk of delivering a baby with low birthweight compared with women with a BMI of 19.8–20.6 (Frederick, Williams, Sales, Martin, & Killien, 2008).

Table 4–1 Recommended Weight Gain Chart

Body Mass Index	Recommended Total Weight
BMI < 19.8	28–40 pounds
Normal BMI (19.8–26.0)	25–35 pounds
Overweight BMI (26.1–29.0)	15–25 pounds
Obese BMI (> 29.0)	15 pounds
Twins	35–40 pounds

Source: CDC, Pediatric and Pregnancy Nutrition Surveillance System. http://www.cdc.gov/pedness/what_is/pnss_health_indicators.htm/maternalheal

RISK FACTORS FOR FETAL GROWTH RETARDATION

The following sections discuss the common risk factors for fetal growth retardation.

Maternal Malnutrition

Malnutrition during pregnancy causes a decrease in placenta blood flow and reduced placenta size, resulting in reduced nutrient transfer to the fetus.

Smoking

A recent study reported by the American Heart Association 2006 Scientific Sessions shows that women who smoke during early pregnancy are 60% more likely to have babies with congenital heart disease than are those who do not smoke. Smoking during pregnancy is associated with infant deaths and increases the risk of cancer during the child's first 7 years of life (Jaakola & Gissler, 2004).

Use of Drugs and Alcohol

Use of illicit drugs and alcohol by pregnant women can harm the fetus. Use of recreational drugs during early pregnancy is a significant risk factor for gastroschisis, according to results of a recent study published in the *American Journal of Epidemiology* (Draper, 2008). Gastroschisis is a rare birth defect in which portions of the intestines of the fetus are found on the outside of the abdomen because of an abnormal opening in the abdominal muscle.

Heavy drinking of alcohol during pregnancy is associated with fetal alcohol syndrome. Major clinical manifestations of fetal alcohol syndrome include birth defects, growth and mental retardation, hyperactivity, problems learning, distractibility, and seizures. The *Journal of the American Academy of Pediatrics* reported a study titled "Binge Pattern of Alcohol Consumption and Childhood Mental Health Outcomes." The study found that occasional episodes of consuming 4 or more drinks per day during pregnancy can adversely affect the child's health, particularly in regard to hyperactivity and inattention problems (Kapil et al., 2009).

Preexisting Medical Conditions and Pregnancy

Diabetes, cardiovascular disease, pulmonary disease, neoplasm, infectious diseases such as HIV/AIDS, and epilepsy can significantly affect fetal growth because of the complications associated with these medical conditions. Close monitoring of the patient including rate of weight gain is extremely important.

Food Intolerance and Allergy

Food allergy and intolerance affect nutrient intake if proper substitutions are not provided. Inadequate nutrient intake impairs fetal growth.

Depression

Depression during pregnancy is quite common. Every year, 1 in 20 American women who are pregnant or who have given birth in the past 12 months suffer from major depression (Jesse, Walcott-McQuigg, Mariella, & Swanson, 2005). Factors associated with depression include hormonal changes, psychosocial instability, inadequate support, presence of a preexisting medical condition such as HIV/AIDS, and a history of depression. Depression during pregnancy can result in delayed prenatal care and poor oral intake, with the risk of permanent damage to the fetus during the first trimester because of inadequate transfer of nutrients via the placenta.

In the absence of adequate treatment, depression can accelerate. Episodes may become more frequent and severe, resulting in substantial maternal and infant morbidity (Bennett, Einarson, Taddio, Koren, & Einarson, 2004).

Although use of medications during pregnancy is usually not recommended, studies have shown that selective serotonin reuptake inhibitors (SSRIs) are relatively safe to use during pregnancy. Nonpharmacologic interventions such as psychotherapy, religion, and education are also helpful.

COMPLICATIONS IN PREGNANCY AND DIETARY INTERVENTION

Nausea and Vomiting

Many pregnant women experience nausea and sometimes vomiting during pregnancy. This is oftentimes referred to as morning sickness. For some women, this occurs in the first trimester; for others, during the entire pregnancy. Nausea and vomiting affect weight gain as a result of inadequate meal consumption. Eating dry crackers or toast with jelly and ginger ale before getting out of bed and limiting fried and greasy food help to relieve nausea. In the case of excessive vomiting with failure to gain weight, nutrition support may be warranted.

Constipation

Constipation is a frequent complaint during pregnancy. Constipation may be the result of iron and calcium supplementation, inadequate fiber and fluid intake, and decreased mobility. Constipation left untreated can lead to fecal impaction. Increased dietary fiber and fluids in addition to daily walks can help to relieve constipation.

Heartburn or Gastroesophageal Reflux Disease (GERD)

Heartburn is estimated to occur in 30–50% of pregnancies, with the incidence approaching 80% in some populations (Richter, 2005). In GERD, the contents of the stomach back up into the esophagus, causing irritation. Patients are encouraged to have small, frequent meals and to sit up for at least 2 hours before lying down. They should avoid greasy and spicy foods, chocolate, spearmint, peppermint, citrus fruits, tomato, and tomato products.

Preeclampsia/Eclampsia

Preeclampsia, also referred to as pregnancy-induced hypertension, is a risk factor for cardiovascular disease. Preeclampsia is a rapidly progressive condition characterized by high blood pressure and the presence of protein in the urine. Swelling, sudden weight gain, headaches, and changes in vision are important symptoms. The cause of preeclampsia remains unknown, but this condition is seen more frequently in first and multiple pregnancies, women older than 35 years of age, obese women, and women with a history of diabetes, high blood pressure and kidney disorder. In preeclampsia, systolic blood pressure is 140 mmHg or higher and diastolic blood pressure is 90 mmHg or higher (Mahan & Escott-Stump, 2008). Eclampsia is preeclampsia accompanied with seizures.

With 3% to 5% of pregnancies complicated by preeclampsia and an average of 128.9 million births per year, approximately 3.87 million to 6.45 million pregnancies per year worldwide are affected by preeclampsia (McDonald, Malinowski, Zhou, Yusuf, & Devereaux, 2008). Preeclampsia can lead to low-birthweight babies, preterm birth, and kidney and liver problems for the mother. A study published in the *New England Journal of Medicine* found no protection against preeclampsia with the use of vitamin C and vitamin E supplementation (Rumbold et al., 2006).

Gestational Diabetes

Diabetes mellitus is one of the most common medical complications of pregnancy; gestational diabetes mellitus (GDM) accounts for approximately 90–95% of all cases. GDM is defined as carbohydrate intolerance of variable severity with onset or first recognition during pregnancy (Menato et al., 2008).

Meeting the nutritional needs of women with gestational diabetes mellitus can be a challenge for dietetics professionals. The main purpose of dietary modification is to maintain normal glucose levels, but this is not the only factor to be considered. You must provide adequate energy to meet the needs of the fetus and achieve an adequate weight gain for the woman. The bottom line is to achieve an optimal outcome for both the infant and the mother (Marcason, 2005).

Following are the risk factors for gestational diabetes mellitus:

- Maternal age older than 30 years
- Obesity
- Family history of diabetes in a first-degree relative
- History of glycosuria
- Elevated blood glucose with previous use of oral contraception
- Previous history of gestational diabetes
- History of pregnancy with stillbirth or babies born weighing more than 9 pounds

Screen women who present with risk factors for GDM for diabetes as you would the nonpregnant woman. Uncontrolled diabetes during pregnancy can lead to neonatal hypoglycemia, hypocalcemia, hyperbilirubinemia, macrosomia (> 4000 g), and respiratory problems. Neonatal hypoglycemia can cause cognitive problems, possible coma, or even death.

Published studies show that after GDM, 10–50% of women develop type 2 diabetes within 5 years (Menato et al., 2008).

Medical nutrition therapy (MNT) is the primary treatment for GDM. The American Diabetes Association recommends the following:

For normal-weight women (BMI 20–25 kg/m²), prescribe 30 kcal/kg. For overweight and obese women (BMI > 24–34 kg/m²), restrict calories to 25 kcal/kg. For morbidly obese women (BMI > 34 kg/m²), restrict calories to 20 kcal/kg or less. Caloric composition includes 40–50% from complex, high-fiber carbohydrates; 20% from protein; and 30–40% from primarily unsaturated fats. The calories may be distributed as 10–20% at breakfast, 20–30% at lunch, 30–40% at dinner, and 30% with snacks, especially a bedtime snack in order to reduce nocturnal hypoglycemia (Menato et al., 2008).

To prevent a rise in blood glucose, breakfast should consist of complex carbohydrates and a source of protein, for example egg or milk. If blood glucose remains uncontrolled even after MNT, add insulin to regimen to better control blood glucose. Increased blood glucose during pregnancy might not always be a result of excess intake of carbohydrates; stress and sickness can also cause a rise in blood glucose.

LACTATION

Breast milk remains the best source of nutrition for the newborn; however, breastfeeding is contraindicated in the presence of the following conditions:

- HIV infection
- Active untreated tuberculosis
- Illicit drug use
- Certain medications such as chemotherapy drugs
- Infants diagnosed with galactosemia

In the absence of the preceding risk factors, encourage the mother to breastfeed. Breast milk contains important antibodies that play a role in protecting the infant's immature gut from infection. It also contains factors that appear to protect the mucosa of the alimentary and respiratory tracts of the infant. Several studies show a positive correlation between breastfeeding and cognitive development.

While lactating, it is important that the mother consumes a balanced diet that provides adequate calories (2500–2800 cal/day) and protein (up to 80g/day). Diet should be rich in calcium, vitamin D, and omega-3 fatty acids. Iron should be about 10 mg/day.

You can also use the questions you use to assess the pregnant woman for postpartum assessment. Asking whether the mother uses drugs and alcohol is always relevant because drugs taken by the mother can be transferred to the infant via breast milk. Address mothers' fears and concerns regarding breastfeeding as well as their cultural view on the subject in the assessment. It is always good to have a nurse or lactation specialist provide instructions to new mothers on latching on, breast engorgement, sore nipples, and other concerns they might have about breastfeeding the baby.

SUMMARY

Careful assessment of the pregnant woman with early dietary intervention is critical to a favorable pregnancy outcome. Poor nutrition, use of drugs, and depression can have life-threatening effects on both the mother and the fetus. It is, therefore, important to monitor the mother's rate of weight gain during pregnancy and provide medical nutrition therapy to address complications associated with pregnancy, including but not limited to gestational diabetes mellitus.

You should carefully screen the lactating mother for proper nutrient intake and instruct her on breastfeeding techniques to ensure that the infant receives adequate amounts of breast milk to facilitate growth.

REVIEW QUESTIONS

1. Sara is a 16-year-old woman who discovered that she is 2 months pregnant. She is 5 ft, 5 in. tall. Weight prior to pregnancy was 115 pounds, BMI 19. She complains of nausea, especially in the mornings. She is no longer attending school.

   a. List all of Sara's nutritional concerns.

   b. Calculate her required caloric intake.

   c. Develop a meal plan to meet Sara's nutritional needs.

2. Jane is a 34-year-old woman who is 3 months pregnant. During the assessment interview, she indicates that her previous child, born in August 2005, weighed 9 pounds, 8 ounces at birth, and that her mother was diagnosed with diabetes 5 years ago.
   a. What would be your concern and why?
   b. What recommendation would you have for Jane at this time?

REFERENCES

Bennett H. A., Einarson A., Taddio, A., Koren, G., & Einarson, T. R. (2004). Depression during pregnancy. *Clinical Drug Investigations, 24*(3), 157–179.

Draper, E. (2008). Recreational drug use in first trimester may increase the risk of gastroschisis. *American Journal of Epidemiology, 167*, 485–491.

Frederick, I. O., Williams, M. A., Sales, A. E., Martin, D. P., & Killien, M. (2008). Pre-pregnancy body mass index, gestational weight gain, and other maternal characteristics in relation to infant birth weight. *Maternal and Child Health Journal, 12*(5), 557–567.

Gautum, C. S., Saha, L., Sekhri, K., & Saha, P. K. (2008). Iron deficiency in pregnancy and the rationality of iron supplements prescribed during pregnancy. *Medscape Journal of Medicine, 10*(12), 283.

Guido, M., Bo, S., Signorile, A., Gallo, M.-L., Cetrino, I., & Botto Poala, C., et al. (2008). Current management of gestational diabetes mellitus. *Expert Review of Obstetrics and Gynecology, 3*(1), 73–91.

Helland, I. B., Smith, L., Saarem, K., Saugstad, O. D., & Drevon, C. A. (2003). Maternal supplementation with very-long-chain n-3 fatty acids during pregnancy and lactation augments children's IQ at 4 years of age. *Pediatrics, 111* (1), e39–e44.

Jaakkola, J. J. K., Gissler, M. (2004). Maternal smoking in pregnancy, fetal development, and childhood asthma. *American Journal of Public Health, 94*, 136–140.

Kapil, S., Heron, J., Golding, J., Alati, R., Smith, G. D., & Gray, R., et al. (2009, February 2). Binge pattern of alcohol consumption during pregnancy and childhood mental health outcomes: Longitudinal population-based study. *Pediatrics, 123*(2), e289–e296.

Javaid, M. K., Crozier, S. R., Harvey, N. C., et al. (2006). Maternal vitamin D status during pregnancy and childhood bone mass at age 9 years: A longitudinal study. *Lancet, 367*, 36–43.

Jesse, E. D., Walcott-McQuigg, J., Mariella, A., Swanson. M. S. (2005). Risks and protective factors associated with symptoms of depression in low-income African American and Caucasian women during pregnancy. *Journal of Midwifery Women's Health, 50*(5), 405–410.

Mahan, L. K., Escott-Stump, S. (2008). *Krause's food, nutrition and diet therapy* (12th ed.). St. Louis, MO: Sanders.

Marcason, W. (2005). What is the appropriate amount and distribution of carbohydrates for a woman diagnosed with gestational diabetes mellitus? *Journal of American Dietetic Association, 105*(10), 1673.

McDonald, S. D., Malinowski, A., Zhou, Q., Yusuf, S., & Devereaux, P. J. (2008). Cardiovascular sequelae of preeclampsia/eclampsia: A systematic review and meta-analysis. *American Heart Journal, 156*(5), 918–930.

Richter, J. E. (2005). Review article: The management of heartburn in pregnancy. *Alimentary Pharmacology and Therapeutics, 22*(9), 749–757.

Rumbold, A.R., Crowther, C.A., Haslam, R.R., Dekker, G.A., Robinson, J.S., & ACTS StudyGroup. (2006). Vitamins C and E and the risks of preeclampsia and perinatal complications. *New England Journal of Medicine, 354*(17) 1796–1806.

State of Connecticut Department of Health. *Diet assessment—Pregnant women. Connecticut WIC Program.*

U.S. Department of Agriculture. (2002). Dietary Reference Intakes: Recommendations for individuals. Food and Nutrition Information Center. Retrieved September 17, 2009, from http://www.iom.edu/Object.File/Master/21/372/0.pdf

U.S. Environmental Protection Agency. (2004, March). *What you need to know about mercury in fish and shellfish.* Retrieved October 1, 2009, from http://www.epa.gov/waterscience/fish/advice/index.html

Pediatric Assessment

ASSESSING THE NEWBORN

In assessing the newborn it is important to understand the meaning of the following terms:

- Normal gestation age (GA): 40 weeks
- Appropriate for gestation age (AGA): Between 10th and 90th percentile
- Small for gestation age (SGA): Percentile < 10%
- Large for gestation age (LGA): Percentile > 90%
- Premature: Gestational age < 38 weeks
- Postmature: Gestational age > 42 weeks
- Macrasomic: Baby > 4000 g
- Low birthweight (LBW): Baby < 2500 g
- Very low birthweight (VLBW): Baby < 1500 g
- Very, very low birthweight (VVLBW): Baby < 750 g
- Failure to thrive: Weight for age < 3rd percentile

NUTRITIONAL CARE OF THE LOW-BIRTHWEIGHT INFANT

Low-birthweight (LBW) infants are babies weighing < 2500 g at birth. Their nutritional needs are great to achieve optimal growth. The LBW infant presents with the following characteristics:

- Minimal energy reserves (both carbohydrate and fat)
- Intrinsically higher metabolic rate (greater relative mass of more metabolically active organs: brain, heart, liver)
- Higher protein turnover rate (especially when growing)
- Higher glucose needs for energy and brain metabolism
- Higher lipid needs to match the in utero rate of fat deposition
- Excessive evaporative rates (immature skin)
- Occasionally very high urinary water and solute losses (depending on intake and renal maturation)
- Low rates of gastrointestinal peristalsis
- Limited production of gut digestive enzymes and growth factors
- Higher incidence of stressful events (hypoxemia, respiratory distress, sepsis)
- Metabolic effects of medications used frequently (steroids, antibiotics, sedatives, catecholamines)
- Abnormal neurologic outcome if not fed adequately (Thureen & Hay, 1993)

The impact of inadequate early nutrition on growth and development of the central nervous system is of particular concern, according to William Heird (1999.) He further states that a large body of data, primarily from animals, but some from human infants, demonstrates that if malnutrition is not corrected during a critical period of brain growth and development, deficits may not be recoupable. In the human infant, this critical period for growth of the entire brain is believed to span at least the first 18 months of life. Thus, correction of early malnutrition before 18 months of age theoretically should circumvent overall deficits (Heird, 1999).

Nutrition Implications and Intervention

To adequately meet the nutritional needs of the LBW infant, initiate nutrition support right after birth, usually in the form of parenteral glucose solutions and progress to parenteral nutrition consisting of glucose, amino acids, electrolytes, and vitamins. Subsequently, provide total parenteral nutrition (TPN) consisting of intravenous glucose, amino acids, electrolytes, vitamins, and lipid emulsions, for maintenance and, if adjusted appropriately, use it to support growth. Minimal enteral nutrition is added to provide small, trophic quantities of milk. As the infant matures physiologically and the medical condition stabilizes, replace TPN slowly with enteral nutrition (Schanler, 1996).

Transitioning very-low-birthweight (VLBW) infants successfully to enteral nutrition is a key to their achieving adequate growth and development without the long-term risks related to parenteral nutrition. Human milk is a key component of any strategy for enteral nutrition of all infants. Its introduction in the first days of life leads to improved growth and better health outcomes for infants (Hawthorne, Griffin, & Adams, 2004).

The energy needs of the growing LBW infant ranges from 100 to 120 cal/kg/day, but can go higher up to 150 cal/kg/day if the infant presents with chronic diseases, such as bronchopulmonary dysplasia, that increase energy requirements because of greater energy expenditure. Protein needs range from 3.0 to 4.0 g/kg/day. Increased protein is important to reverse the negative nitrogen balance characteristic of the first days after birth, increase the serum concentration of amino acids, and increase the rate of protein synthesis (Hay, 2008).

Table 5–1 compares the nutritional needs of the term infant with the preterm infant. Calcium and phosphorus are needed in adequate amounts to reduce the risk of bone undermineralization, fractures and rickets, which may result from inadequate intakes of calcium and phosphorus.

Weigh LBW infants at the same time each day, and measure length and head circumference weekly. Biochemical monitoring is also done weekly.

Table 5–2 compares suggested nutrient and energy intake for parenteral and enteral nutrition for LBW infants.

Oral Feeding for the Low-Birthweight Infant

Assess the infant for feeding readiness. In an article published in *Neonatal Network*, McCain (2003) states that "the ability of a preterm infant to make the transition from gavage to oral nipple feeding depends on the infant's neurodevelopment in relation to behavioral organization, to a

Table 5–1 Daily Requirements of Selected Nutrients in Healthy Term and Preterm Infants

Nutrient	Normal Requirements	
	Term[a]	Preterm
Energy		
Total (kcal/kg)	100	120
Carbohydrate (g/kg)	10	12 to 14
Fat (g/kg)	3.3 to 6	4 to 7
Protein (g/kg)	1.5 to 2.2	3.0 to 4.0
Minerals and Trace Elements		
Sodium (mEq/kg)	1 to 3	2 to 4
Potassium (mEq/kg)	1 to 2	2 to 4
Calcium (mg/kg)	45 to 60	120 to 230
Orthophosphate (mg/kg)	25 to 40	60 to 140
Magnesium (mg/kg)	6 to 8	7.9 to 15
Iron (mg/kg)	1[b]	2 to 4[b]
Vitamins		
A (IU/kg)	333	700 to 1,500
E (IU)	3 to 25	5 to 25

[a] Based on infants fed human milk.
[b] Iron supplementation starts at 2 weeks postnatal age.
Source: Heird, William, C. *The Importance of Early Nutritional Management of Low-birthweight Infants.* Pediatrics in Review, 20, 43–43, 1999 © American Academy of Pediatrics.

rhythmic suck-swallow-breathe pattern, and to cardiorespiratory regulation" (p. 45).

Breast milk is usually the food of choice for the newborn, but fortification may be needed to adequately meet the demands of the LBW infant. A study reported in the *Minerva Pediatrica* states that, although some nutrients are initially increased in the milk of mothers delivering prematurely, there are inadequate amounts of calcium, phosphorus, zinc, and other nutrients to meet the needs of the VLBW infant during growth. Therefore, safe and effective means of fortifying human milk are essential to the care of VLBW infants (Hawthorne et al., 2004).

Infants with slow growth and infants in whom biochemical abnormalities or impaired nutritional status have been identified may require an

Table 5-2 Comparison of Suggested Parenteral and Enteral Fluid, Energy, and Nutrient Intake for LBW Infants

Component (units)	Parenteral Intake (unit/kg/d)	Enteral Intake (unit/kg/d)
Water (mL)	150	150
Energy (kcal)	80–100	120–130
Protein (g)	3.0–3.5	3.5
Fat (g)	1.0–4.0	5.0–7.0
Carbohydrate (g)	16	12.0–14.0
Vitamin A (IU)	500	700–2000
Vitamin D (IU)	160	400
Vitamin E (IU)	2.8	5–25
Vitamin K (µg)	80	7–9
Thiamine (vitamin B_1) (µg)	350	20–40
Riboflavin (vitamin B_2) (µg)	150	60
Pyridoxine (vitamin B_6) (µg)	180	35–60
Vitamin B_{12} (µg)	0.3	0.1–0.5
Niacin (mg)	6.8	0.8
Folic acid (µg)	56	50
Sodium (mEq)	2.0–4.0	2.0–8.0
Potassium (mEq)	2.0–3.0	2.0–3.0
Chloride (mEq)	2.0–3.0	2.0–3.0
Calcium (mg)	80–120	200–220
Phosphorus (mg)	60–90	100–110
Magnesium (mg)	9–10	7–10
Zinc (µg)	350–450	1000–2000
Copper (µg)	65	65–300
Chromium (µg)	0.4	0.1–0.4
Manganese (µg)	10	7.5
Selenium (µg)	2.0	1.0–2.0

Source: Schenler, R. L. (1996). The Low-birthweight Infant. In W. A. Waller & J. B. Watkins (Eds.), *Nutrition in pediatrics—basic science and clinical application* (2nd ed., pp. 393–407). Hamilton, Ontario: BC Decker.

enriched milk after hospital discharge. To provide this nutrition you can add a standard formula diluted to 24 kcal/oz to alternate with breastfeeding or by using 24 kcal/oz formula exclusively (Schanler, 1996). Formula must be rich in the essential fatty acids—linoleic acid, linolenic acid, and arachidonic acid. Essential fatty acids are needed for optimal neurodevelopment and to prevent dermatitis and stunted growth.

ASSESSING THE FULL-TERM INFANT

The full-term infant has a gestational age of 40 weeks. The expected daily weight gain is shown in **Table 5–3**. **Table 5–4** shows the calorie and protein requirements for children, from infancy to age 10 years. See **Figure 5–1** and **Figure 5–2** for length-for-age and weight-for-age percentiles for girls and boys from birth to 36 months.

FAILURE TO THRIVE

Not all full-term babies develop as expected. Delay in weight gain could be caused by prematurity, the presence of an illness, inadequate nutrient intake secondary to poor feeding technique, cultural barriers, health beliefs, social and psychological problems in the family, poverty, a strict diet, severe food allergy, vomiting, diarrhea, dysphagia, infections, adenoid hypertrophy, and respiratory problems such as bronchopulmonary dysplasia. All of these risk factors can result in what is called "failure to thrive," where the weight for age is < 3rd percentile.

Both weight and head circumference are measured and plotted on the growth chart to determine proper postnatal growth. Consider the growth

Table 5–3 Expected Daily Weight and Monthly Height Gain of Infants and Young Children

Age	Grams/day	Centimeters/month
0–3 months	20–30	2.6–3.5
3–6 months	15–20	1.6–2.5
6–12 months	10–15	1.2–1.7
1–6 years	5–8	0.5–1.1
7–10 years	5–11	0.4–0.6

Table 5–4 Calorie and Protein Requirements of Infants and Young Children

Age	Calories per Kilogram	Grams of Protein per Kilogram
0–6 months	108	2.2
6–12 months	98	1.6
1–3 years	102	1.2
4–6 years	90	1.1
7–10 years	70	1.0

Note: Fluid requirement is approximately 100 mL/kg/day.

of other siblings and the stature of the parents when evaluating an infant or child with growth failure. Look at the growth history to determine appropriate weight gain or growth failure. Your assessment of the child with failure to thrive must include the medical history, prenatal history, events at birth, for example, prematurity, congenital malformation and infections, social and family history, as well as gastrointestinal review. **Table 5–5** lists the Waterlow criteria for determining malnutrition (Duggan, 1997, p. 705–713).

According to the Waterlow criteria, chronic malnutrition refers to height for age, whereas acute malnutrition looks at weight for height. The percentage of the median is determined by the following equation:

$$\% \text{ Median} = \frac{\text{Actual weight} \times 100}{\text{Median weight}}$$

where median weight is the median value for age and sex (Duggan, 1997).

Nutritional Implications and Intervention

The infant who presents with malnutrition is at high risk for cognitive and developmental delays. Malnutrition is also associated with poor performance in school. The child who presents with growth delay needs additional calories and protein. Calories must be adequate so that protein stores are not used for energy.

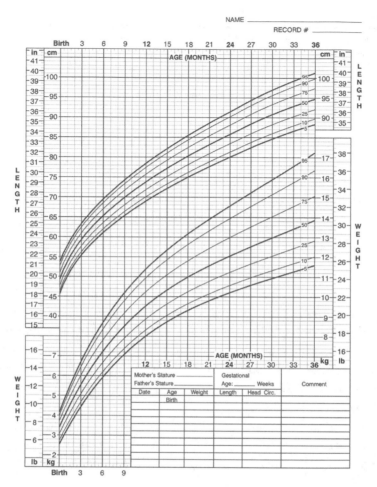

Figure 5-1 Birth to 36 Months: Girls Length for Age and Weight for Age Percentiles

Source: Developed by the National Center for Health Statistics in collaboration with the National Center for Chronic Disease Prevention and Health Promotion (2000). http://www.cdc.gov/growthcharts

To achieve catch-up growth to correct growth deficiency, use the following guideline:

$$\text{Kcal per kg required} = \frac{\text{RDA for age (kcal/kg)} \times \text{Ideal weight for height}}{\text{Actual weight}}$$

where ideal weight for height is the median weight for the patient's height, obtained from weight for height growth chart. Use the same formula to determine protein requirement.

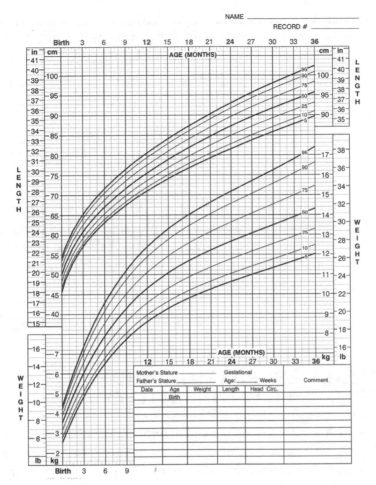

Figure 5-2 Birth to 36 Months: Boys Length for Age and Weight for Age
Percentiles

Source: Developed by the National Center for Health Statistics in collaboration with the
National Center for Chronic Disease Prevention and Health Promotion (2000). http://www
.cdc.gov/growthcharts

Example: SJ is a 5-month-old boy with a length of 58 cm and weight
of 4.5 kg. His caloric requirement for catch-up growth is as follows:

RDA for age is 108 cal/kg.

His ideal weight for height is 5.5 kg.

Required calories/kg: 108 × 5.5 / 4.5 = 132 kcal/kg

Be sure to address the etiology of the poor nutrient intake, whether it is
medical or socioeconomic. Iron-deficiency anemia in infants and preschool

Table 5–5 Waterlow Criteria for Acute and Chronic Malnutrition

	Acute (weight for height) (% of median)	Chronic (height for age) (% of median)
Normal	> 90	> 95
Mild	80–90	90–95
Moderate	70–80	85–90
Severe	< 70	< 85

children results in developmental delays and behavioral disturbances. Increasing the strength of the formula can provide additional calories. For older children, adding extra margarine, olive oil, cheese, and milk powder to food can help increase calories. Snacks such as ice cream, peanut butter, sherbet, cakes, and cookies can also be included in the diet.

Children presenting with food allergy should be given suitable substitution to meet dietary needs. See Chapter 2 for information on food allergy and how to read food labels.

MENTAL RETARDATION AND DEVELOPMENTAL DISABILITY

Children with mental retardation and developmental disability are at risk for obesity, chronic constipation, and osteoporosis caused by limited mobility. Some anticonvulsant medications predispose patients to constipation. Dysphagia is quite common in severe mental retardation, so a diet of modified consistency is required for easy swallowing. Thickened fluids are sometimes offered while aspiration precaution is maintained for all meals.

Drooling, or sialorrhea, is common in children with moderate to severe cerberal palsy. This may occur as a result of hypersecretion of saliva, low oral muscle tone with poor lip closure, inadequate jaw control, postural problems, inability to recognize salivary spill, and dental malocclusion (Wilson-Jones, Morgan, & Shelton, 2007). Drooling, though a risk factor for dehydration, is also a good indicator of adequate hydration in the patient with cerebral palsy.

For patients with severe dysphagia, enteral nutrition is the primary source of nutrition.

The caloric requirement for children with developmental delays is different from that of children of similar age because of their limited activity. Caloric requirements are based on calories per centimeter of height. **Table 5–6** outlines caloric recommendations for children with developmental delays.

INBORN ERRORS OF AMINO ACID METABOLISM

Inborn errors of amino acid metabolism are metabolic disorders that impair the synthesis and degradation of amino acids. These disorders include but are not limited to homocystinuria, phenylketonuria, and maple syrup urine disease, which are discussed in the following subsections.

Homocystinuria

Homocystinuria is an autosomal recessive disorder caused by a deficiency of cystathionine beta-synthase that results in high plasma concentrations of methionine and homocysteine with elevated excretion of homocysteine in the urine. Normal levels of homocysteine are 5.90–16 micromol/L. Homocystinuria caused by cystathionine beta-synthase deficiency affects at least 1 in 200,000 to 335,000 people worldwide (U.S. National Library of Medicine, 2008).

Table 5–6 Estimated Energy Needs for Children With Developmental Delays

Condition	Daily Caloric Recommendation
Ambulatory, ages 5 to 12 years	13.9 kcal/cm height
Nonambulatory, ages 5 to 12 years	11.1 kcal/cm height
Cerebral palsy with severely restricted activity	10 kcal/cm height
Cerebral palsy with mild to moderate levels of activity	15 kcal/cm height
Down syndrome, boys ages 5 to 12	16.1 kcal/cm height
Down syndrome, girls ages 5 to 12	14.3 kcal/cm height

Source: Courtesy of Duggan, C. (1996). Failure to thrive: Malnutrition in the pediatric outpatient setting. In W. A. Walker & J. B. Watkins (Eds.), *Nutrition in pediatrics—basic science and clinical application* (2nd ed., pp. 705–714). Hamilton, Ontario: BC Decker.

Clinical manifestation of the disease includes detached retina, abnormal blood clots, skeletal abnormalities, and mental retardation. Skin manifestations include malar flush, thin hair, and cutis reticulata/marmorata (Rao, Rahakrishna, Mohana Rao, Guruprasad, & Ahmed, 2008). Patients may also experience weakness of the muscles of the pelvic girdle and a shuffling gait.

Pyridoxine (vitamin B_6) has proven helpful in managing the disease. For patients who respond well to pyridoxine therapy a normal but not excessive protein intake is recommended. For those who do not respond well to pyridoxine therapy, a low-protein diet or methionine-free formula with added L-cysteine is used. Hominex is one such formula produced by Abbott Nutrition. Diet should provide adequate calories from carbohydrate and fat to meet the nutritional needs of the patient.

Phenylketonuria

Phenylketonuria (PKU) is the most common inborn error of amino acid metabolism. It is caused by a deficiency of phenylalanine hydroxylase, which normally converts phenylalanine to tyrosine. Phenylalanine can build up to harmful levels in the blood, and if this condition is not treated early can cause developmental delay or even severe mental retardation. Skin disorders, musty odor, and seizure disorders are some of the clinical manifestations of the disease.

A diet low in phenylalanine starting in the first month of life can significantly reduce mental retardation, the most important feature of the disease. For infants and children, a phenylalanine-free formula is provided, supplemented with regular infant formula or breast milk during infancy and cow's milk in early childhood to provide high-biologic-value protein, nonessential amino acids, and sufficient phenylalanine (Phe) to meet the individualized requirements of the growing child (Trahms & Ogota, 2008). Tyrosine is also added to the formula. Low-protein pasta, cereal, and baked products can offer variety to the diet.

Maple Syrup Urine Disease

In maple syrup urine disease (MSUD), also known as branched chain ketoaciduria, an oxidative decarboxylase in the white blood cells is missing. Because the carboxyl group cannot be removed, the three branched-chain amino acids (BCAs), leucine, isoleucine, and valine, and their corresponding ketoacids and L-hydroxyacids build up in the blood and are excreted in excessive amounts in the urine. The urine has a sweet-smelling odor similar to that of maple syrup.

Infants appear normal at birth, but begin to show symptoms within the first few days of life. They are unable to suck and swallow satisfactorily, respiration is irregular, and they exhibit intermittent periods of rigidity and flaccidity. Seizures may be present. Failure to treat MSUD can result in neurologic deterioration, seizures, coma, and eventually, death. MSUD presents with life-threatening cerebral edema and dysmyelination in affected individuals. Treatment requires lifelong dietary restriction and monitoring of BCAAs to avoid brain injury (Zinnanti et al., 2009).

The goal of treatment is to maintain a diet low in leucine, isoleucine, and valine. The blood concentrations of these amino acids are carefully monitored. Specialized formula low in BCAAs and containing other essential amino acids is offered to promote normal growth and development in the patient with MSUD.

EATING DISORDERS IN CHILDREN AND ADOLESCENTS

Eating disorders are complex disorders involving two sets of issues and behavior: those directly relating to food and weight, and those involving the relationship of oneself with others (American Dietetic Association, 2006). Eating disorders fall into three main categories: anorexia nervosa, bulimia nervosa, and binge eating disorder. The following subsections discuss the diagnostic criteria for each as outlined by the American Psychiatric Association.

Anorexia Nervosa

Patients with anorexia nervosa exhibit the following behaviors:

- Refusal to maintain body weight at or above a minimally normal weight for age and height (e.g., weight loss leading to maintenance of body weight less than 85% of that expected; or failure to make expected weight gain during period of growth, leading to body weight less than 85% of that expected)

- Intense fear of gaining weight or becoming fat even though underweight
- Disturbance in the way in which one's body weight or shape is experienced, undue influence of body weight or shape on self-evaluation, or denial of the seriousness of the current body weight (American Psychiatric Association, 1994)

Bulimia Nervosa

Bulimia nervosa is recurrent episodes of binge eating. An episode of binge eating is characterized by both of the following features:

- Eating in a discrete period of time (e.g., within any 2-hour period) an amount of food that is definitely larger than most people would eat during a similar period of time and under similar circumstances
- A sense of lack of control over eating during the episode (e.g., a feeling that one cannot stop eating or control what or how much one is eating)

The patient also exhibits recurrent inappropriate compensatory behavior to prevent weight gain, such as self-induced vomiting; misuse of laxatives, diuretics, enemas, or other medications; fasting or excessive exercise.

The binge eating and inappropriate compensatory behaviors both occur on average at least twice a week for 3 months (American Psychiatric Association, 1994).

Binge Eating Disorder

Binge eating disorder is recurrent episodes of binge eating. An episode of binge eating is characterized by both of the following features:

- Eating in a discrete period of time (e.g., within any 2-hour period) an amount of food that is definitely larger than most people would eat during a similar period of time and under similar circumstances and
- A sense of lack of control over eating during the episode (e.g., a feeling that one cannot stop eating or control what or how much one is eating)

The binge eating episodes are associated with at least three of the following conditions:

- Eating much more rapidly than normal
- Eating until feeling uncomfortably full
- Eating large amounts of food when not feeling physically hungry
- Eating alone because of being embarrassed or feeling very guilty after overeating

The binge eating is not associated with the regular use of inappropriate compensatory behaviors (e.g., purging, tasting, excessive exercise) and does not occur exclusively during the course of anorexia nervosa and bulimia nervosa (American Psychiatric Association, 1994).

All three eating disorders have serious medical and nutritional implications, and although they begin with preoccupations with food and weight, they are most often about much more than food. Psychological factors that can contribute to eating disorders are feelings of low self-esteem, inadequacy, depression, anxiety, anger, or loneliness. Interpersonal factors such as problems with family or other relationships, difficulty expressing emotions and feelings, being ridiculed or teased based on size or weight, and a history of sexual abuse are factors associated with eating disorders (National Eating Disorders Association, NEDA,1998). Chemical imbalance in the brain is being investigated as a possible contributory factor to eating disorders. Society places pressure on young people to be thin, and it defines beauty as being of a certain body size.

The following are some questions that you can use to identify eating disorders in adolescents. The list is by no means exhaustive.

- Do you avoid foods containing a lot of sugar or fat?
- Are you terrified of gaining weight?
- Does it take you longer than others to complete your meal?
- What portions of your meal do you tend to eat or not eat?
- Do you think you are preoccupied with reading food labels and counting calories?
- Do you eat a lot of diet foods?
- Do you exercise a lot, especially after eating a meal?
- Do you avoid eating even when you are hungry?
- Do you feel guilty after eating food?

- Do you feel the need to vomit after eating?
- Do you feel that food controls your life?
- Do you feel that family and friends pressure you to eat?

Treating eating disorders requires a multifactorial approach and involves the primary care physician, psychotherapist, psychiatrist, and nutritionist. Interactive individual and group counseling along with family involvement and support help to achieve success in patients with eating disorders.

Nutritional Implications and Intervention

Eating disorders can have serious long-term medical consequences including cardiac problems, kidney failure, and eventually death. Malnutrition associated with anorexia nervosa can affect nearly every organ system in the body, with cardiac complications responsible for 50% of the deaths in anorexia nervosa (Tamburrino & McGinnis, 2002).

Binge eating disorder is associated with obesity and can lead to diabetes, high blood pressure, and cardiac problems later on.

Reduced fluid intake, frequent vomiting, and frequent bowel movement resulting from the abuse of laxatives can lead to dehydration and low blood pressure.

Amenorrhea (no menstrual period) is associated with anorexia nervosa and results from a lack of body fat and too much rigorous exercise. Inadequate intake of food leads to stunted growth, constipation, osteopenia, iron-deficiency disease, edema caused by low protein stores, and electrolyte imbalance.

To treat patients with eating disorders, be sure to be knowledgeable about the psychological aspects of eating disorders. Nutrition goals must be realistic, and involve the patient in creating goals. Nutrition treatment goals for anorexia nervosa, typically referred to as nutritional rehabilitation, relate to restoration of a healthful weight and normalization of eating patterns. Make gradual adjustments in nutrient intake and weight progress such as stepping up calorie intake from a baseline level of between 30 and 40 kcal/kg/day of actual weight per day (may start at 1000 to 1200 kcal per day). Incremental advancement to achieve a weight gain of 0.5 to 1.0 lb per week may be attainable—even for patients with chronic conditions (American Dietetic Association, 2006).

Set a weight goal of 90–110% of ideal body weight. Be patient, caring, and nonjudgmental, and be a good listener. Achieving caloric goals takes time, so small, frequent feedings are advised. Meals for patients with eating disorders should be calorically dense and balanced. Increased protein intake is necessary to correct edema. Fluids must be adequate for electrolyte balance. A multivitamin/mineral supplement is usually prescribed.

PEDIATRIC OBESITY

Childhood obesity is on the rise. At the Environmental Public Health Leadership Institute, Werner von Kutzleben (2007) reported that in 2004 the World Health Organization (WHO) estimated that 1 in 10 children worldwide was overweight, or more than 22 million children under the age of 5. The WHO considers obesity to be one of the 10 causes of preventable deaths and the result of a worldwide nutrition transition, which is reflected in profound lifestyle and behavioral changes within society.

Weight gain during childhood is attributed to poor eating habits, sedentary lifestyle, cultural values, and socioeconomic status. It is a fact that high-calorie foods and snacks are cheaper than healthful foods. The increase in the number of fast-food restaurants offering low-cost high-calorie foods contributes to the increase in weight in children and adolescents—portions are huge and high in calories. Consumption of soda is high among children whereas intake of milk is low. **Figure 5–3** and **Figure 5–4** show the body mass index-for-age percentiles for girls and boys.

Nutritional Implications and Intervention

Not only do overweight and obese young people face major health consequences of diet-related chronic diseases such as type 2 diabetes, cardiovascular disease, hypertension, high blood pressure and cholesterol levels, sleep apnea, and premature death, but they also must cope with a reduction in the quality of life and experience social stigmatization and discrimination. The latest study from the Centers for Disease Control and Prevention estimates that about 112,000 deaths are associated with obesity each year in the United States (CDC, Press Release, 2005). New

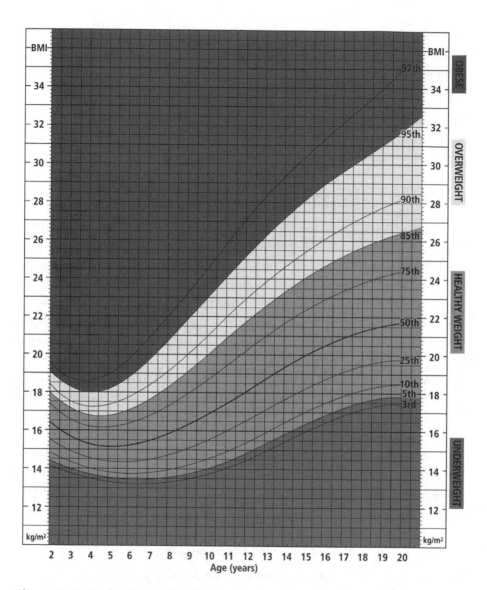

Figure 5–3 Body Mass Index-for-Age Percentiles Girls

Source: Adapted from the Centers for Disease Control and Prevention (CDC) Growth Chart New York State Department of Health.

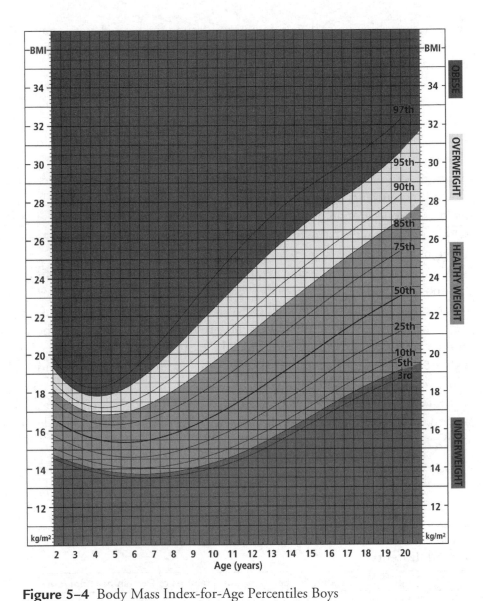

Figure 5–4 Body Mass Index-for-Age Percentiles Boys

Source: Adapted from the Centers for Disease Control and Prevention (CDC) Growth Chart New York State Department of Health.

research shows that more than 6 million children in the United States may have nonalcoholic fatty liver disease, especially those who are overweight or obese (Schwimmer, 2006).

In treating obesity in children, you must be sensitive to the child's feelings and provide support in making lifestyle changes. As with eating disorders, family involvement is crucial to achieving any level of success. Family history and cultural values must be explored. Explain to the child that there are no "bad" foods, but that some foods provide very little health benefit and predispose one to weight gain, while other foods provide lots of nutrients to help the body grow healthy. Always have available pictures of food or food models. Help the child set goals for healthy food selections and physical activity. For example, set a goal such as "eat three different fruits this week."

Many children eat fast foods frequently. Encourage the family to limit fast foods and to consider preparing foods at home. On days when they order out, teach parents and children how to make healthier selections. Restaurants and fast-food establishments are now mandated to post the number of calories for each food item in clear view of the customer. **Table 5–7** lists calorie and protein requirements for older children and adolescents.

Review the Food Guide Pyramid and Activity Pyramid with families as a good way to get parents and children thinking about healthy lifestyle changes.

Table 5–7 Nutritional Requirements for Older Children and Adolescents

	Age	Calories per Kilogram	Grams of Protein per Kilogram
Males	11–14 years	55	1.0
	15–18 years	45	0.9
Females	11–14 years	47	1.0
	15–18 years	40	0.9

SUMMARY

Achieving and maintaining adequate nutrition in infants and children are important to facilitate proper growth and development. Growth failure must be investigated and addressed aggressively to prevent serious complications later in life. Being sensitive to the feelings of children and adolescents in treating eating disorders and obesity can help facilitate healthy lifestyle changes.

REVIEW QUESTIONS

1. Xavier is a 3-month-old boy who weighs 3.6 kg. His length is 57 cm. Calculate his caloric requirements for catch-up growth.
2. Jane is a 7-year-old girl with mental retardation and developmental delay. Her length is 80 cm. She is nonambulatory and has severe dysphagia. Calculate her caloric requirements. What would be a suitable diet for this patient?

REFERENCES

American Dietetic Association. (2006, December). Nutrition intervention in the treatment of anorexia nervosa, bulimia nervosa, and other eating disorders. *Journal of the American Dietetic Association, 106*(12), 2073–2082.

American Psychiatric Association. (1994). *Diagnostic and statistical manual of mental disorders* (4th ed.). Washington, DC: Author.

Centers for Disease Control and Prevention. (2005, June 14). *CDC's National leadership role in addressing obesity* [press release]. Retrieved October 5, 2009, from http://www.cdc.gov/media/pressrel/r050615.htm

Duggan, C. (1996). Failure to thrive: Malnutrition in the pediatric outpatient setting. In W. A. Walker & J. B. Watkins (Eds.), *Nutrition in pediatrics—basic science and clinical application* (2nd ed., pp. 705–714). Hamilton, Ontario: BC Decker.

Hawthorne, K. M., Griffin, I. J., & Abrams, S. A. (2004). Current issues in nutritional management of low birth weight infants. *Minerva Pediatrics, 56*(4), 359–372.

Hay, W. W., Jr. (2008). Strategy for feeding the preterm infant. *Neonatology, 94*(4), 245–254.

Heird, W. C. (1999). The importance of early nutritional management of low birth weight infants. *Pediatrics in Review, 20*, 43–44.

McCain, G. C. (2003). An evidence-based guideline for introducing oral feeding to healthy preterm infants. *Neonatal Network, 22*(5), 45–50.

Mahan, L. K., & Escott-Stump, S. (2008). *Krause's food and nutrition therapy,* (12th ed.). St. Louis, MO: Sanders.

National Eating Disorders Association (NEDA). (1998). *Causes of eating disorders.* Retrieved October 5, 2009, from http://www.nationaleatingdisorders.org/information-resources/general-information.php#causes-eating-disorders

Premer, D. M., & Georgieff, M. K. (1999). Nutrition for ill neonates. *Pediatrics in Review, 20,* 56–62.

Rao, T. N., Radhakrishna, K., Mohana Rao, T. S., Guruprasad, P., & Ahmed, K. Homocystinuria due to cystathionine beta synthase deficiency. (2008). *Indian Journal of Dermatology, Venereology, and Leprology, 74*(4), 375–378.

Schanler, R. J. (1996). The low birth weight infant. In W. A. Walker & J. B. Watkins (Eds.), *Nutrition in pediatrics—basic science and clinical application* (2nd ed., pp. 393–407). Hamilton, Ontario: BC Decker.

Schwimmer, J. (2006). National digestive diseases information clearinghouse: Nonalcoholic steatohepatitis. *Pediatrics, 118,* 1388–1393.

Tamburrino, M. B., & McGinnis R. A. (2002). *Anorexia nervosa. A review. Panminerva Medica, 44,* 301–311.

Thureen, P., & Hay, W. W., Jr. (1993). Conditions requiring special nutritional management. In R. C. Tsang (Ed.), *Nutritional needs of the preterm infant.* Baltimore: Williams & Wilkins.

Trahms, C. M., & Ogata, B. N. (2008). Metabolic nutrition therapy for genetic metabolic disorders. In L. K. Mahan & S. Escott-Stump (Eds.), *Krause's food and nutrition therapy* (12th ed., pp. 1141–1157). St. Louis, MO: Saunders.

U.S. National Library of Medicine. (2008, October 30). *Homocystinuria.* Retrieved October 5, 2009, from http://ghr.nlm.nih.gov/condition=homocystinuria

von Kutzleben, W. (2007–2008). *The childhood and adolescent obesity epidemic confronting Virginia schools, 2007–2008.* Environmental Public Health Leadership Institute. Retrieved September 17, 2009, from http://www.cdc.gov/nceh/ehs/EPHLI/reports/vonkutzeleben.doc

Walker, W. A., & Watkins, J. B. (Eds.). (1996). *Nutrition in pediatrics—basic science and clinical application* (2nd ed.). Hamilton, Ontario: BC Decker.

Wilson Jones, M., Morgan, E., & Shelton, J. E. (2007). Primary care of the child with cerebral palsy: A review of systems (part II). *Journal of Pediatric Health Care, 21*(4), 226–237.

Zinnanti, W. J., Lazovic, J., Griffin, K., Skvorak, K. J., Paul, H. S., Homanics, G. E., et al. (2009). Dual mechanism of brain injury and novel treatment strategy in maple syrup urine disease. *Brain 132*(4), 903–918.

Solving the Problem

Creating a Plan of Care

Determining Nutrient Requirements and Writing the Care Plan

After you have collected all the evidence from the chart, patient interview, observation, and analysis using various assessment tools, you can identify the patient's problem and provide a solution for that problem. Once a nutrition problem or diagnosis is identified in the second step of the Nutrition Care Process, the next step is to design a plan to provide intervention to address that nutritional diagnosis. This chapter focuses on the third step in the Nutrition Care Process—nutrition intervention.

The Nutrition Care Process dictates that nutrition intervention consists of two interrelated components: planning and intervention. Planning involves prioritizing diagnoses based on urgency, impact, and available resources; collaborating with the patient to identify goals; and writing a nutrition prescription based on the patient's needs, health condition, and nutrition diagnosis. Implementation of the nutrition intervention involves communicating the plan of care and collaborating with the patient or caregiver to carry it out. You may also need to revise the plan of care based on changes in the patient's condition or his or her response to intervention.

The patient's caloric and protein requirements are determined by the following factors, most of which are discussed in earlier chapters:

- Age and gender
- Body weight, height, and composition
- Activity level
- Medication effects (see Table 1–4)
- Presence and severity of illness
- Infection and fever
- Malabsorption
- Current oral intake
- Abnormal nutrition-related laboratory values
- Trauma and wounds
- Pregnancy
- Lactation

Table 6–1 provides recommendations for calories and protein for patients with common diseases and medical conditions that warrant nutrition intervention. Values are based on ideal body weight (IBW).

DETERMINING FLUID NEEDS

Fluid balance is evaluated by the presence of edema, changes in skin turgor, intake/output, the osmolality of serum and urine. Fluids needs are increased in the presence of an infection, evidenced by increased temperature and also when the patient shows signs of dehydration. Signs of dehydration include foul-smelling urine; sunken eyes; dry/chapped lips; elevated blood urea nitrogen (BUN), sodium, chloride, and glucose; restlessness or delirium; headache; tachycardia; decreased skin turgor; and low blood pressure. An increased albumin level in a patient with poor oral intake is also a sign of dehydration. A weight loss of 1 kg is equivalent to 470 mL of water.

Fluid needs are estimated at 30–35 mL/kg of body weight using actual body weight. Fluid needs for obese individuals are calculated at 30–35 mL/kg of ideal body weight.

Some conditions such as congestive heart failure and kidney disease require a reduction in fluids to maintain optimal health. Reduction of fluid is important especially for patients on dialysis. Daily fluid needs for dialysis patients are usually determined by the nephrologist and range

Table 6-1 Determining Calorie and Protein Needs

Category of Activity or Illness	Kcal/Kg/Day	Grams Pro/Kg/Day
Minor surgery	30 cal/kg	1.0–1.2 g/kg
Major surgery	35 cal/kg	1.5–2.0 g/kg
Major sepsis	40–45 cal/kg	1.5–2.0 g/kg
Peritonitis	35–40 cal/kg	1.2–1.4 g/kg
Trauma, for example, severe burns	40–45 cal/kg	1.5–2.0 g/kg
Malnutrition with starvation	20–22 cal/kg	1.1–1.5 g/kg
Significant weight loss	30–35 cal/kg	1.2–1.5 g/kg
Crohn's disease	30–35 cal/kg	1.0–1.2 g/kg
Acute renal insufficiency	30–35 cal/kg	0.8–1.0 g/kg
Chronic kidney disease w/o dialysis	35 cal/kg	1.0 g/kg
Chronic kidney disease w/ hemodialysis	35 cal/kg	1.2–1.4 g/kg
Chronic kidney disease w/ peritoneal dialysis	25–30 cal/kg	1.2–1.5 g/kg
Diabetes type I, II	30 cal/kg	0.8–1.0 g/kg
Paraplegia	28 cal/kg	0.8–1.0 g/kg
Quadriplegia	23 cal/kg	0.8–1.0 g/kg
AIDS	35 cal/kg	1.2–1.5 g/kg
AIDS, with wasting syndrome	40–50 cal/kg	1.5–2.0 g/kg
Hepatic disease, cirrhosis	30–35 cal/kg	1.2–1.5 g/kg
Hepatic disease with encephalopathy	30–35 cal/kg	0.8–1.0 g/kg
Acute pancreatitis	35–40 cal/kg	1.2–1.5 g/kg
Chronic pancreatitis	30–35 cal/kg	1.0–1.2 g/kg
ICU patients on ventilator	25 cal/kg	1.2–1.4 g/kg
Geriatrics	25–30 cal/kg	1.0–1.1 g/kg
Pregnancy, using prepregnant IBW	36 cal/kg	1.0–1.2 g/kg
Pneumonia	30–35 cal/kg	1.0–1.5 g/kg
Pulmonary failure, if catabolic	35–40 cal/kg	1.5–2.0 g/kg
Cancer, if severely stressed	35–40 cal/kg	1.5–2.0 g/kg

from 1000 mL to 1500 mL fluid per day. Excess fluids in these patients can result in shortness of breath, high blood pressure, edema, ascites, hyponatremia, and subsequent death. Fluid gain between dialysis treatments is carefully monitored and the patient is educated on how to be compliant with fluid restriction.

Fluid needs for the patients who are tube fed are usually 1 mL/cal (Charney & Malone, 2009). Calculations of fluids include water from formula as well as free water used for flushes and medications. Evaluate patients often for signs of hyponatremia and fluid overload. Signs of over-hydration include increased blood pressure, decreased pulse rate, edema, azotemia, change in mental status such as restlessness, and decreased sodium, chloride, albumin, creatinine, BUN, hematocrit, hemoglobin, and potassium (Doenges, Moorhouse, & Murr, 2008).

CREATING A PLAN OF CARE

After you have decided on a solution to the problem affecting the nutritional status of the patient, the next step is to create a plan of care to address the problem. **Table 6–2** presents a sample care plan. Each identifiable problem must have a care plan. Note, however, that care plans are used mainly in long-term care facilities and are hardly ever used in a hospital setting.

Quality indicators that must be addressed in documentation are the following:

- Weight loss
- Fecal impaction
- Prevalence of tube feeding
- Prevalence of parenteral nutrition
- Hydration/dehydration
- Pressure sores
- Fluid restriction for dialysis patients
- Education and teaching

Fecal impaction and dehydration are sentinel events, the prevalence of which can cause a facility to lose Medicare/Medicaid dollars and possibly be subject to closure. Although some medical conditions predispose patients to dehydration, you must clearly document intervention to prevent such an event and evaluate the outcome.

The **care plan** should include the following items:

- The nutrition-related problem
- Goals for the patient
- Intervention

Table 6–2 Sample Care Plan

Date	Problem	Goal	Intervention	Target Date	Responsible Disciplines	Outcome
06/12/08	Significant wt loss of 6% in 1 month	To gain 1–5 pounds	Provide Ensure Plus 8 oz PO (2 × day) Add extra margarine to lunch and dinner	09/08	✔ Nursing ✔ Dietary ✔ MD	Achieved _____
06/12/08	Poor oral intake— consumes < 50% of meals	To achieve oral intake of 75–100%	Provide Megace as ordered Honor food preferences Monitor food intake for ≥ 75% Monitor weight monthly	09/08	✔ Activity	Continue thru _____ Discontinued because _____

Source: Split Rock Nursing Home and Rehab Center.

- Outcome evaluation (answers the questions, "Was the goal met? Why or why not?")
- Disciplines responsible for achieving goals
- The date the plan was developed
- The date the goal(s) was/were written
- Target date for the goal

Writing Goals

Following are some general guidelines on how to write effective goals.

- Goals must be specific and measurable. Goals must address the specific problem and be applicable to the disease state, for example. weight loss, low albumin, poor oral intake, or anemia. Goals must be measurable, for example, "Patient will gain 1–5 pounds," instead of "Patient will increase weight." If a patient is edematous and has poor oral intake, instead of weight gain, a reasonable goal would be for the patient to meet 75–100% of her caloric/protein needs. If a patient has a low serum albumin of 3.0 g/dL, a reasonable measurable goal would be "Patient's albumin will improve > 3.0 g/dL."
- Goals must be time sensitive. State the target date for the achievement of the goal, for example, "Patient will gain 1–5 pounds in 3 months, or by October 2008." If a goal is not met as expected, set a new target date to achieve the goal.
- Goals must be achievable. The patient is the central focus of the care plan and should be included in the goal-setting process. Listen carefully to the patient's concern and assess learning readiness to help facilitate compliance in achieving goals. For example, an achievable goal is "to lose 1–5 pounds in 3 weeks."
- Always date changes. If a specific change has to made to a written goal, date the change and set a new target date for achieving the goal. Discontinued goals must be dated as such with a note stating why the goal was discontinued, for example, "goal met," "patient transferred to another facility," or "patient expired."

Intervention/Recommendation

Nutrition intervention is found in the plan section of the assessment as well as in the care plan. It must be clear, precise, and specific. It is best to list recommendations using numbers or bullets. Physicians usually look at the Plan section of the assessment to determine the next step in treating the patient, especially if a nutrition consult was ordered.

Always provide supporting evidence when making recommendations, for example, the nutrition plan might read, "recommending Ensure Plus 8 oz 2 × day due to significant weight loss and poor oral intake" (indicate the percentage of weight loss over a specified period of time in the assessment).

Note the type and frequency of nutritional supplementation. Do the same for tube feeding; state the name of the formula, the amount of the formula, the amount and frequency of free water flushes, the rate of feeding, the route of feeding, the duration of the feed, and the calories and protein provided by the formula. Always indicate the reason for recommending tube feeding. For example, "Recommending 1600 mL Probalance at 100 mL/hr via PEG for 16 hours, providing 1920 calories, 86 g protein. Flush with 200 mL water every shift." (Please note that this rate is not recommended for patients who are just starting tube feeding.)

Should you decide to recommend an appetite stimulant to improve oral intake, documentation must be in place to show actual intake of meals and supplements in terms of percentage over a period of time. Never specify the type of appetite stimulant to be given because some medications might interact with others and cause an adverse reaction. For example, Periactin (cyproheptadine HCl) should not be used with other antihistamines such as Benadryl (diphenhydramine). The physician will decide on the drug of choice.

Monitoring Procedures

Nutrition monitoring and evaluation identifies the amount of progress made and whether goals/expected outcomes are being met. Information is gathered to determine reasons for lack of progress or to identify other problems or negative outcomes.

Monitoring procedures, where applicable, must also be included in the care plan. If a patient is new to tube feeding, you must monitor for signs/symptoms of aspiration, discomfort, bloating, high residuals, constipation, diarrhea, and vomiting. Other monitoring procedures might include monitoring weight weekly, biweekly, or monthly; monitoring specific labs, for example, blood glucose in diabetes and patients new to tube feeding; triglycerides, especially in the administration of total parenteral nutrition (TPN); and monitoring oral intake, if any, based on set goal(s). Fluid intake and an output record are usually kept for the patients who tube feed.

The standards of practice for nutrition support are divided into five areas: assessment, therapeutic plan, implementation, patient monitoring, and transitional feeding. Established criteria are used to identify a patient who is or may become malnourished, and provision is made for nutrition support based on the patient's nutritional needs and clinical status. A nutrition care plan is developed and the clinical and metabolic response to nutrition support is monitored to provide a basis for modifying nutrition support therapy (Winklers, 1993).

It might also be necessary to monitor the frequency and give a description of bowel movements in patients who are constipated or having diarrhea. Always follow up on the intake of nutritional supplements to determine the effectiveness of the intervention.

Transitioning to Oral Feeding

Before a patient on tube feeding can be considered for oral feeding, the speech-language pathologist must be consulted for a swallow evaluation. Once the speech-language pathologist agrees that the patient can start oral feeding, give small amounts of pureed snacks, for example, pudding or plain yogurt. Make no change to tube feeding at this time.

Carefully document tolerance of snack items and the amount given and percentage consumed in the patient's medical record. If there are no complications with the pureed snacks, after two days introduce one meal (breakfast, lunch, or dinner), preferably at a time when tube feeding is not being administered. Then, calculate the caloric and protein intake of the meal consumed.

Offer the same meal for about three days, and if the patient's intake is consistent or increases, decrease the tube feeding based on the calories consumed from the meal/snack. Repeat this pattern for the remaining two meals, each time reducing the tube feeding by the number of calories consumed until the patient is able to meet his or her caloric needs with oral feeds only. Document adequacy of intake before discontinuing parenteral or enteral nutrition support (Winklers, 1993). If oral nutrient intake is suboptimal, do not discontinue enteral nutrition (American Society for

Parenteral and Enteral Nutrition and the Standards for Specialized Nutrition Support Task Force, et al., 2005).

Some patients will continue to do well on oral feeds after being weaned from tube feeding, but some patients' condition will decline, causing poor oral intake and a return to tube feeding. Ongoing monitoring of caloric intake is necessary to ensure that nutritional status is not compromised.

Outcome Evaluation

Outcome evaluation is step 4 of the Nutrition Care Process. Outcome indicators must be relevant to the nutrition diagnosis or its signs or symptoms, nutrition goals, and medical diagnosis. Outcomes must be measured against appropriate reference standards. This section of the Nutrition Care Process seeks to explain variance from expected outcomes and determine factors that help or hinder progress (Writing Group of the Nutrition Care Process/Standardized Language Committee, 2008).

In the outcome evaluation, you look at whether the goal has been met and evaluate the need to revise the goal. Once the goal is met, it should be discontinued with the date inserted in the care plan.

Evaluating the outcome of your intervention proves your worth as a dietitian and shows your importance to the healthcare team. It shows how you help save healthcare dollars through medical nutrition therapy.

If a patient is receiving nutritional supplement for weight gain, assess the patient for continuation or discontinuation of the supplement once the target goal is reached. If oral intake is good on solid foods, and the weight goal is met, reduce and subsequently discontinue supplements. If a supplement has to be continued because of fluctuating intake, documentation should be in place to justify the need to continue use of the supplement.

Follow-up Plans

Proper follow-up is extremely important in the delivery of nutrition care. Follow-up plans may include referral to another discipline to address a certain deficiency, for example, the speech-language pathologist for a swallow evaluation or occupational therapist to evaluate the use of utensils and positioning. Inform the relevant clinician in a timely manner and document the referral in the medical record accordingly after informing the other clinician. Some facilities require the person making the referral to complete a requisition form, a copy of which goes to the clinician who is responsible for the evaluation.

Follow-up plans may also include revisiting a particular issue within a given time frame. Always be realistic with follow-up plans so as to be in compliance and not appear negligent. If your plan is to follow up on weight monthly, do this monthly. If you document that diet teaching will follow, do the teaching as stated.

Education and Teaching

Nutrition intervention must include education and teaching. If teaching is not feasible because the patient has dementia or anoxic encephalopathy, indicate this on the care plan. Always determine the patient's level of knowledge and priority of learning needs so as to make each teaching session precise and easily understood. Always include a returned demonstration, for example, "JB was able to identify three food items high in potassium."

If family members are present for assessment or follow-up, educate them on the nutrition intervention *only* if they are listed as a proxy for that patient. Always keep the patient's information confidential. Only those who are listed as proxies should be given information regarding the patient's medical status. If the patient and the spouse/family members are present for teaching, document this on the education sheet. **Table 6–3** shows a sample patient education record.

Documentation of patient teaching must include the patient's response to the teaching. Words used to describe the response are:

receptive
not receptive
asks questions
receptive but needs reinforcement
denial of diagnosis
verbalized understanding
returned demonstration with assistance
returned demonstration independently

Always document what you actually taught the patient; be specific and do not generalize.

Table 6–3 Sample Patient Education Record

Topics	Readiness	Barriers	Taught to Whom	Methods	Outcomes	Evaluation
1. Medications 2. Disease 3. Equipment 4. Community resources 5. Nutrition 6. Food/drug interaction 7. ADL 8. Tests and procedures 9. Advance directives 10. Other	1. Asks questions 2. Eager to learn 3. Unreceptive 4. Declines instruction 5. Denies need	1. Language 2. Cultural 3. Religious 4. Cognition 5. Reading 6. Hearing 7. Vision 8. Emotional 9. None	1. Resident 2. Spouse 3. Significant other 4. Parent 5. Son/daughter 6. Caregiver	1. One on one 2. Group session 3. Audio/visual 4. Demonstration 5. Phone contact 6. Handout	1. Verbalized understanding 2. Returned demonstration 3. Returned demonstration with assistance 4. Refused to learn 5. Unable to learn	1. No further teaching required 2. Reinforce content 3. Needs practice 4. Reteach 5. Seek additional support
Topic 6 Specify **low-Na food choices**	**Number** 2	**Number** 9	**Number** 1, 2	**Number** 1	**Number** 1, 2	**Number** 3
Date 9/10/08	**Signature** *Miriam Black*		**Credentials** RD, CDN	**Title** Dietitian		**Department** Food/Nutrition

Note: ADL = activity of daily living.

Source: Bronx Lebanon Special Care Center.

If you gave handouts to the patient, note this on the education sheet. The education sheet is multidisciplinary and should be completed each time a patient is educated on any condition related to his or her health. The format varies among facilities.

Discharge Instructions

If a patient is being discharged from the hospital/nursing home, patient teaching must be done and the patient must be informed of referrals in the community, for example, following up with an outpatient dietitian for control of hyperglycemia. Always provide a contact number where the patient can reach you or another dietitian should the individual have any questions regarding diet after discharge.

Patients who have diabetes but do not have a glucometer must be provided with one before discharge. The social worker is usually involved to ensure that the patient gets this device before leaving the facility. Document returned demonstration using the glucometer. This function is usually performed by the nurse, but you must teach the signs and symptoms of hypoglycemia and hyperglycemia, carbohydrate substitution, and how to treat hypoglycemia should blood glucose fall below 70 mg/dL, or 80 mg/dL for some patients. Patients who have had a history of hyperglycemia will experience symptoms of low blood glucose at or below 80 mg/dL. Do not overwhelm patients with lengthy handouts. Keep information short and simple.

Patients who are discharged on tube feeding must be instructed on proper handwashing techniques to minimize the risk of infection and contamination, especially with bolus feeding. Further details are provided in Chapter 8, "Diet Teaching for Specific Medical Conditions."

SUMMARY

The care plan gives a clear description of the problem(s) being addressed by the dietitian and the intervention to meet set goals. Care plans should be reviewed periodically. Most institutions review them every quarter and reevaluate and update goals. Monitoring procedures are important to determine the success of an intervention.

REVIEW QUESTIONS

1. JB was admitted to your facility today from the hospital with poor PO intake and weight loss of 7% over the last 4 weeks. Dx: AIDS with wasting syndrome. Labs indicate Alb 2.1. What would be a suitable goal(s) for this patient?
2. You received a medical consult for the reintroduction of oral foods for a patient who is on enteral tube feeding. What steps would you take for possible weaning from enteral nutrition? What other disciplines would be involved to facilitate the process?

REFERENCES

American Society for Parenteral and Enteral Nutrition Board of Directors and the Standards for Specialized Nutrition Support Task Force, et al. (2005). Standards for specialized nutrition support: Home care patients. *Nutrition in Clinical Practice 20*(5), 579.

Charney, P., & Malone, A. M. (2009). *ADA pocket guide to nutrition assessment* (2nd ed.). Chicago, IL: American Dietetic Association.

Doenges, M. E., Moorhouse, M. F., & Murr, A. C. (2008). *Nursing diagnosis manual: Planning, individualizing and documenting client care* (2nd ed.). Philadelphia, PA: F. A. Davis.

Winklers, M. (1993). Standards of practice for the nutrition support dietitian: Importance and value to practitioners. *Journal of the American Dietetic Association 93*(10), 1113–1118.

Writing Group of the Nutrition Care Process/Standardized Language Committee. (2008). Nutrition care process and model part I: The 2008 update. *Journal of the American Dietetic Association, 108*(7), 1113–1117.

ADDITIONAL RESOURCES

American Dietetic Association. *Nutrition care manual.* http://www.nutritioncaremanual.org.

Emery, E. A. (2007). Nutrition diagnosis and intervention: A case report. *Journal of the American Dietetic Association 107*(8), A22.

Heimberger D. C. & Ard, J. (2006). *Handbook of clinical nutrition* (4th ed.). St. Louis, MO: Mosby, Inc.

CHAPTER 7

Patient Teaching

E ducating patients on their medical conditions is extremely important to ensure the success of nutrition intervention and a desirable outcome. Careful assessment of the patient prior to teaching is critical because it saves time and reduces frustration. Use the medical chart to get information on the patient that can help you formulate an appropriate teaching strategy. The patient's willingness to learn might be influenced by his or her religious beliefs; physical condition, for example, the presence of pain; physical limitation such as deafness; visual impairment; language barrier; intellectual abilities; and learning styles (McVan & Cahill, 1987).

Consider the following factors when developing teaching strategy for your patient:

1. *Cognition of the patient.* Cognition is the ability to think and solve problems. Impaired cognition in adults may be associated with seizure disorder, multiple sclerosis, Parkinson's disease, traumatic brain injury, stroke, brain tumor, dementia, or Alzheimer's disease. Impaired cognition results in short-term memory problems, poor problem-solving skills, and an impaired ability to conceptualize.

Cognitive abilities decline with age. The decline is slow and gradual. Older adults, therefore, need more time to learn new skills.

Individuals with cognitive impairment usually are not auditory learners; therefore, teaching must be geared toward showing rather than telling. Have the patient repeat tasks several times until he grasps it, before moving to a new task or concept. Use short, direct sentences and hands-on approaches when providing diet instructions. Always offer lots of positive feedback to help boost the patient's confidence.

2. *Level of literacy.* It is important to determine the patient's literacy level before attempting to teach about diet and the patient's health. One study of patients found that average word recognition skill was four to five grades lower than the level of schooling declared by patients. Patient education pamphlets usually require an eighth-grade reading level; oral instructions are frequently presented at a tenth-grade level or higher (Chatham & Knapp, 1982).

To reach the patient with low literacy, use information and language that has been simplified to ensure comprehension, compliance, and cooperation. Chatham and Knapp (1982) suggest the following techniques:

- Speak (write) in short sentences, conveying no more than one concept per sentence.
- Speak (write) words that have few syllables; one- or two-syllable words are best.
- Speak (write) words that are meaningful to the patient, not technical or uncommon to the average lay person.
- Speak (write) in a conversational active voice, for example, "do fingersticks just before eating breakfast and at 8 pm before going to bed" instead of "do fingersticks twice a day."

Effective teaching strategies for patients with low literacy include the following:

- Returned demonstration
- Two-way conversation
- Use of food models and realistic photos
- Repetition of instruction and concepts

- Posing open-ended questions to evaluate learning, for example, "Mr. Brown, let's say you checked your blood sugar and the result was 60. What would you do?"

3. *Resources available to the patient.* Officially, in the United States, the working poor are defined as individuals who spent at least 27 weeks in the labor force (working or looking for work), but whose income fell below the official poverty level. Since the start of the recession in December 2007, the number of unemployed persons has increased by 7.6 million to 15 million, and the unemployment rate has doubled to 9.2 percent (Bureau of Labor and Statistics, 2009). Limited access to nutritious food constitutes food insecurity.

   It is estimated that as many as 3.5 million people are homeless over the course of a year. Three percent report having HIV/AIDS, and 26% report acute health problems other than HIV/AIDS such as tuberculosis, pneumonia, or sexually transmitted diseases. Some studies indicate that the prevalence of HIV among homeless people is as high as 20%. Even higher prevalence rates (8.5–62%) have been reported in various homeless subpopulations, including adults with severe mental illness. Of the 400,000 to 600,000 individuals currently estimated to be living with AIDS in the United States, approximately one third to one half are either homeless or at imminent risk of homelessness (National Prevention Information Network, n.d.).

   Homelessness is associated with poor health. Many working poor depend on food pantries and soup kitchens for a hot meal. Resources are limited, and purchasing nutritious foods is not always on their priority list. Foods offering little nutritional value are less expensive than healthy foods are. The emergency room serves as the primary care physician for many working poor and homeless persons.

   Given the limited resources of some patients, it is imperative that diet instructions be simple and affordable and offer no more than two dietary changes that the patient can accommodate. Focus your instruction on the area of priority that poses the highest nutrition risk and incorporate the patient's usual activities. When instructing the patient who is homeless or who has limited access to nutritious food, include in the plan prepackaged nutritious and ready-to-eat foods that need no preparation as many homeless persons have no access to a cooktop or oven to prepare their meals. Refer patients to social services or other community resources for follow-up to help meet their financial needs.

4. *Patient's willingness to modify behavior.* The Transtheoretical Model, also referred to as the Stages of Change Model, describes a five-stage temporal process by which people make behavior changes (Nothwehr, Snetselaar, Yang, & Wu, 2006). The stages are as follows:

   a. Precontemplation stage. Not intending to change behavior in the foreseeable future.

   b. Contemplation stage. Intending to change behavior in the next 6 months.

   c. Preparation stage. Intending to change behavior in the immediate future.

   d. Action stage. Overt changes in behavior have been made within the past 6 months.

   e. Maintenance stage. Attempting to avoid relapse but less actively engaged in change processes.

Motivational interviewing has been used by health professionals to promote health behavior changes and help individuals increase their motivation or "readiness" to change. It is a directive, client-centered counseling style that helps clients explore and resolve ambivalence (Flattum, Friend, Neumark-Sztainier, & Story, 2009).

You must assess the patient's stage of change to plan for effective intervention to move the patient to the next level of change. As you question the patient to determine her willingness to change, you must listen carefully to her fears and concerns, which will greatly affect the desired outcome.

Always ask open-ended questions. For example:

"So, tell me, what do you fear most about having diabetes?"
"What do you miss most, now that you have to follow a special diet for diabetes?"

Follow-up questions about the patient's fears might include something like this:

"If I hear you correctly, you are saying that sticking your finger in the mornings hurts, and you would rather not do it?"

Once you have identified the patient's fear/concern, educate the patient on the importance of the change and the detriment associated with non-compliance. Give options or alternatives that will foster adherence. Always find out from the patient what he is willing to do to effect the change before ending the interview.

WRITING LEARNING OBJECTIVES

Learning objectives are statements written to guide the teaching activities of the educator in terms of teaching methods and content to be taught. They state the expected patient results and provide a means for you to measure and evaluate the patient's progress.

Objectives must be simple and centered on the learner. Use an action verb and assign a single task to be completed by the patient, for example:

1. Patient will be able to **name** three food items that are high in potassium.
2. Patient will be able **explain** the difference between saturated fats and unsaturated fats.
3. Patient will be able to **identify** foods high in carbohydrates.

Other action verbs appropriate for learning objectives are *state, describe, define, demonstrate, perform, list, use*, and *test*. The teaching plan should have no more than three objectives to ensure success and compliance.

EVALUATING PATIENT TEACHING

Evaluation is an integral part of the teaching process and must be given consideration prior to teaching the subject. To evaluate patient teaching, examine whether the objectives were met and the effectiveness of the teaching method. If the objectives were not completely met, evaluating the outcome tells what progress was made, if any, and indicates the need to reassess the teaching method and the patient's learning readiness. Be sure to look for barriers that may have hindered patient learning and whether changes have occurred in terms of patient knowledge, skills, attitude, and practices. Evaluation can occur during the teaching session and does not necessarily have to occur at the end of a session.

Evaluating the educator allows the educator to improve in his or her teaching skills. It looks at strengths and weaknesses, effectiveness of teaching method(s), time frame of presentation, patient/family satisfaction, clarity of presentation, organization, and sequence of presentation (McVan & Cahill, 1987).

The patient, family, and/or professional peers can evaluate you, the teacher. Self-evaluation is also an important tool. It is said that "you have not taught until the student has learned." Learning, in almost all cases, relates to a change in behavior.

Evaluation Methods

You can use various methods to evaluate efficacy of teaching. Sometimes more than one method is used. Following are some evaluation techniques:

- *Questioning (interview).* With this method of evaluation, ask the patient questions about the subject to be taught or what is being taught, for example, "What do you know about high blood pressure?" or "What can occur as a result of high blood pressure?" Reword questions as needed to ensure that the patient understands the question you are asking. Present questions in terms clearly understood by the patient.
- *Direct observation.* This method is often referred to as return demonstration, where the teacher observes the patient demonstrating a skill that has been taught. Direct observation provides immediate feedback and actively involves the patient. Human beings remember 90% of what they say and do. Having the patient select foods high in a particular nutrient or low in fat and cholesterol is an example of direct observation.
- *Simulation method.* With this method of evaluation, you present a scenario to the patient and ask how she would handle the situation. Simulation allows the patient to apply skills and knowledge that she has learned in real-life situations. For example, you might say to the patient, "You checked your blood sugar, and it is 55 mg/dL. What would you do?" If the patient answers correctly by saying that she would drink some juice, you might continue by saying, "How much would you drink, and how soon after drinking the juice do you check your blood sugar again?"
- *Written tests.* Pre- and posttests are commonly used to determine learning. Use the same questions before and after the teaching

session. Written tests are a useful tool for teaching large groups; however, they work only with patients who are literate. Questions must be without ambiguity and should focus on the main points to be covered and then covered in the presentation. Keep questions to a minimum and vary them from easy to more difficult.

Multiple-choice format is commonly used in pre- and posttests but can be difficult to construct. Answers should not follow a set pattern, for example, when all the correct answers happen to be letter B. The same holds true for true and false questions. Always vary the correct response so that a pattern is not obvious.

- *Checklists.* Checklists are simple and quick. They list specific activities that the patient should have mastered in the teaching session. They show what goals were achieved and what goals need further work. Here is an example:

Yes	No	Low Fat/Low Cholesterol Education
☐	☐	Identifies the milk lowest in fat and cholesterol
☐	☐	Identifies two suitable low-fat cooking methods
☐	☐	Identifies three foods high in fiber
☐	☐	Identifies three foods high in fat and cholesterol

The following strategy was used by the Memorial Sloan-Kettering Cancer Center in New York to help improve patient education:

a. Computer-generated lists were used to identify new admissions and their prescribed diets.

b. Patients received initial individualized quick-read Diet Information Cards upon admission, which were distributed with their first meals by tray delivery staff.

c. Dietitians followed up with in-depth instructions and detailed diet-specific educational materials packaged in custom-colored envelopes titled "Your Special Restricted Diet."

d. Patients' comprehension was assessed by asking two or three diet-specific questions after instructions. Daily meal rounds provided further opportunities to reinforce instructions (McLymont, Apicello, & Okada, 2006).

As a result of the improved education strategy, Memorial Sloan-Kettering's Press Ganey scores showed significant improvement, averaging 80.4, and placing them at the 99th percentile.

The goal of nutrition education is to convey information in such a way that it is easily understood and can effect behavioral change.

SUMMARY

Helping patients make healthful changes is the goal of medical nutrition therapy. Changes, however, are dependent on the patient's willingness and readiness to change. Asking the right questions prior to the teaching session helps you to learn more about the learner as well as how to formulate effective teaching strategies to meet learning objectives.

REVIEW QUESTIONS

1. Sam Brown has been living on the streets for the past 6 months. His main meal for the day is taken at a shelter in his neighborhood. He was rushed to the hospital after collapsing at the shelter. He was diagnosed with diabetes mellitus. You received a medical consult to counsel this patient. What would be your teaching strategy?
2. Formulate an evaluation tool for the patient Sam Brown in question 1.

REFERENCES

Chathman, M. A., & Knapp, B. L. (1982). *Patient education handbook.* Bowie, MD: Robert J. Brady.

Flattum, C., Friend, S., Neumark-Sztainier, D., & Story, M. (2009). Motivational interviewing as a component of a school-based obesity prevention program for adolescent girls. *Journal of the American Dietetic Association 109*(1), 91–94.

McLymont, V. E., Apicello, A., & Okada, T. (2006). Improving patient satisfaction in nutrition education. *Journal of the American Dietetic Association 106*(8), A47.

McVan, B. & Cahill, M. (1987). *Patient teaching (Nurse's reference library).* Springhouse, PA: Springhouse Publisher.

National Prevention Information Network. (n.d.). The homeless. Retrieved September 17, 2009, from http://www.cdcnpin.org/scripts/population/homeless.asp

Nothwehr, F., Snetselaar, L., Yang, J., & Wu, H. (2006). Stage of change for healthful eating and use of behavioral strategies. *Journal of the American Dietetic Association 106*(7), 1035–1041.

Diet Teaching for Specific Medical Conditions

In the following table, you can find essential information that you should teach to patients diagnosed with specific medical conditions. You might not be able to incorporate all areas in a single teaching session; follow-up sessions may be needed to achieve learning goals. Remember the KISS rule: "Keep it short and simple." Diet teaching is included in step 3 of the Nutrition Care Process that focuses on intervention.

Medical Condition	What to Teach
Hypertension	**Sodium intake.** Increased sodium intake has been linked to high blood pressure. There is a strong correlation between sodium intake and fluid retention. Review with the patient foods high in sodium and the importance of reading food labels. Monosodium glutamate (MSG) found in some cooking spices should be avoided. Encourage use of herbs for flavoring.

The danger of uncontrolled high blood pressure. High blood pressure can lead to damage to the eyes, kidneys, brain as in a stroke, heart, and possibly death.

Normal blood pressure reading. Ideal blood pressure is < 130/80 mmHg, especially for people with diabetes. Blood pressure should be checked frequently because patients might exhibit no symptoms, which is why high blood pressure is sometimes referred to as the "silent killer."

Compliance with medications. Antihypertensive medications are used to keep blood pressure under control and should be taken as prescribed. High blood pressure cannot be cured, it can only be controlled. Reducing or discontinuing medication without a doctor's consent can lead to severe rebound hypertension (McVan & Cahill,1987).

Physical activity. Being physically active helps to maintain normal blood pressure. Weight loss should be encouraged in the patient who is overweight. Excess weight puts more pressure on the cardiovascular system, thereby increasing blood pressure. Encourage aerobic exercise. Some patients will need medical clearance for strenuous activities.

Smoking. Nicotine causes arterioles to constrict, thereby increasing blood pressure. Encourage smoking cessation.

Stress. Reducing stressful conditions can significantly reduce high blood pressure. A good support system is important in managing stress. Adequate sleep, meditation, exercise, taking slow and deep breaths, and taking a vacation are some ways to relieve stress. |
| Hyperlipidemia | **Different type of fats.**

Saturated Fats: Sources and Their Effect on the Heart
Saturated fats are found in whole milk, butter, meat, skin of poultry, cheese, coconut, and coconut oil and can cause fatty deposits along the walls of the arteries, thereby increasing the risk of coronary artery disease. Saturated fats have a tendency to raise blood cholesterol.

Unsaturated Fats
Unsaturated fats are classified as monounsaturated fatty acids and polyunsaturated fatty acids. Monounsaturated fatty acids are found in olive oil, canola oil, peanut oil, pecans, almonds, peanuts, and avocado and have a protective effect on the heart. Polyunsaturated fatty acids can be found in vegetable oils (omega-6) and fish oils (omega-3). Fish oils tend to lower cholesterol. |

Medical Condition	What to Teach

Hyperlipidemia (continued)	**Trans Fats**
	
	Trans-fatty acids are produced when hydrogen is added to harden unsaturated oils. They are found mainly in stick margarine, shortening, baked products, and commercial fats used for frying. Some data suggest that increased intake of trans fats is associated with coronary artery disease.
	
	Dietary cholesterol and triglycerides. Cholesterol is found in animal products. Shrimp, though low in fat, is high in cholesterol. Limit egg yolks to three per week.
	
	Goals:
	  a. Total cholesterol: < 200 mg/dL
	  b. LDL: ≤ 100 mg/dL
	  c. HDL: Men > 40 mg/dL
	             Women > 50 mg/dL
	  d. Triglycerides: < 150 mg/dL
	
	Ways to improve lipid profile:
	• Increase soluble fiber.
	• Make lifestyle changes—smoking cessation, weight loss.
	• Exercise, which helps to increase HDL. Encourage walking; strenuous activities require medical clearance.
	• Choose foods low in saturated fats/cholesterol.

Congestive Heart Failure	**Explain what congestive heart failure (CHF) is.** CHF occurs when the heart loses its ability to act as a pump, resulting in decreased blood flow to the rest of the body. **Complications associated with CHF.** • Pulmonary edema • Thromboembolism (blood clots) • Pedal edema • Mental confusion and memory loss • Damage to kidneys and liver **Strict adherence to diet and medications.** Follow a low-sodium diet. Increased sodium intake can exacerbate CHF by causing fluid accumulation, which in turn increases hypertension and forces the already-compromised heart to work harder. It is important to take medication as prescribed to prevent decompensation. Small, frequent meals are better than large ones. Fluid restriction is not necessary except as recommended by physician. **Medications that affect potassium level.** Lasix (furosemide) causes loss of potassium, whereas Aldactone (spironolactone) can cause an increase in potassium level. Review high-potassium foods with the patient. **Activity.** Overexertion can put more pressure on the heart. Adequate rest is recommended. Walking is encouraged and can be increased gradually; however, if shortness of breath or fatigue is evident, then patient must rest.

(continues)

Medical Condition	What to Teach
Chronic Kidney Disease (on dialysis)	**Functions of the kidney.** The kidney is responsible for the production of red blood cells, removing waste from the body, keeping bones healthy, maintaining growth and blood pressure, and regulating water homeostasis. **Consequences of kidney failure.** • Buildup of waste products • Anemia • Brittle bones • Fluid accumulation (edema, ascites) • Hyperkalemia, which can lead to cardiac arrest • Hyperphosphatemia, which can affect the bones, making them weak • Hypercalcemia, which can cause calcium deposits in soft tissues **Explanation of diet.** *Sodium.* Excess sodium intake will result in fluid accumulation, which in turn can cause an increase in blood pressure. Review with patient high-sodium foods to avoid. *Phosphorus.* A buildup of phosphorus in the blood leads to loss of calcium from the bones. Review phosphorus content of common foods and the importance of taking phosphorus binder as prescribed with meals. *Potassium.* High levels of potassium can lead to an irregular heart rate and subsequent cardiac arrest. Review with patient foods high in potassium. *Protein.* Protein intake must be adequate to ensure good nutritional outcome because protein is often lost during dialysis treatment. BUN > 50 is indicative of adequate protein intake. *Fluids.* The physician will prescribe the amounts of fluids the patient will need. Explain to the patient the reason for the restriction of fluids: the damaged kidneys cannot get rid of excess fluids, and with fluid accumulation there is high risk of increased blood pressure, shortness of breath, swelling to lower extremities, and ascites. Review with the patient what is considered a fluid and how to manage fluids and relieve mouth dryness. Patients may use frozen fruits, sour candies, crushed ice, and lemon wedges, and sip instead of gulping to control fluid intake. *Calories.* Adequate caloric intake is important so that protein is not used for energy. Increase carbohydrates. If the patient has diabetes, follow a diabetes meal plan that provides adequate carbohydrates and protein.

Medical Condition	What to Teach
Chronic Kidney Disease (not on dialysis)	All of the preceding instructions apply, except for protein intake. The protein intake for the patient not yet on dialysis should be limited because of high blood urea nitrogen (BUN). Protein intake should be of high biological value—eggs, meat, chicken, fish, dairy. Encourage the patient to have smaller portions of these products.
HIV/AIDS	**Nutritional complications associated with HIV/AIDS:** • Chronic fatigue • Oral candidiasis • Weight loss • Diarrhea **Nutritional implications of antiretroviral medications:** • Lypodystrophy (fat redistribution) • Hyperlipidemia and increased risk for coronary artery disease (CAD) • Anemia • Osteopenia/osteoporosis • Insulin resistance • Liver damage (hepatotoxicity) • Formation of kidney stones (Bartlett & Gallant, 2005–2006) **Dietary management.** Increase intake of protein, calories, and dark green leafy vegetables. Ensure adequate intake of calcium-rich foods. In the presence of hyperlipidemia, follow a low-fat, low-cholesterol diet with high fiber intake. Utilize nutritional supplements to prevent weight loss. Increase intake of fluids and fiber to aid diarrhea. Provide foods and fluids adequate in potassium to replace lost electrolytes. **Food safety:** Shopping Safely Do not purchase foods past the expiration date on the label. Keep cold and frozen foods separate from the rest of the groceries. Do not purchase foods with damaged or torn packages. Make sure eggs are not cracked or dirty. Purchase only refrigerated eggs. Hot foods purchased outside the home should be consumed soon after purchase. Proper Storage of Food Refrigerate or freeze foods as soon as possible after buying them. Thaw foods in the microwave or in the bottom of the refrigerator, not on the kitchen counter. Refrigerate leftovers in small quantities in airtight containers soon after cooking and use in 1–2 days.

(continues)

Medical Condition	What to Teach
HIV/AIDS (continued)	**Food Preparation** Wash hands thoroughly before and after handling foods. Sanitize cutting boards and counters with a mixture of 1 tsp bleach to 1 gallon of warm water. Wash all fruits and vegetables with water and lemon juice. Cook meats and poultry to > 165° F—there should no sign of blood when cooked. Do not eat foods containing raw egg. Cooked eggs should not be runny, but opaque and firm. Cutting boards used for raw meat, poultry, and seafood should not be used for vegetables and other ready-to-eat foods (Food Marketing Institute, 1996). **Lifestyle changes:** • Exercise • Smoking cessation • Weight loss for those who are overweight • Adherence to therapeutic diet for hypertension, diabetes, hyperlipidemia • Abstaining from illicit drugs
Diabetes	**Etiology of the disease.** Diabetes occurs when the body does not produce enough insulin, as in type 1 diabetes, or the body cannot use well the insulin it produces, as in type 2 diabetes, causing an increase of sugar in the blood. Insulin, oral medication, diet, and exercise can help to control the sugar levels. **Consequences of uncontrolled blood sugar.** Uncontrolled blood sugar can affect the heart, kidneys, eyes, feet, and nerves, and delays the healing of wounds. Can cause sexual impotence. **Signs and symptoms of hyperglycemia.** These include hunger, increased thirst, urination, dry itchy skin, blurred vision. **Signs and symptoms of hypoglycemia.** These include dizziness, sweating, fatigue, blurred vision, irritability, increased anxiety, trembling, and feeling cold, clammy, and nervous. May feel very hungry. **Acceptable values for pre-meal and 2 hours post-meal:** Before meal: 90–130 mg/dL 2 hours after: ≤ 180 mg/dL Bedtime: ≤ 160 mg/dL **Importance of glucose monitoring.** Checking blood sugar with a glucometer at least twice a day lets the physician and other healthcare personnel know how well the medication or insulin is working. Patients should take a reading 2 hours after a meal as well as before a meal. It is important that the patient keeps a record of fingersticks. Most glucometers store the values for a number of days. Patients should be encouraged to bring the glucometer when visiting the doctor or dietitian.

Medical Condition	What to Teach
Diabetes (continued)	**Treating low blood sugar (hypoglycemia).** If blood sugar falls below 70 mg/dL, treat with ½ cup juice or regular soda or 3 glucose tablets and recheck in 15 minutes. If blood sugar does not increase, repeat the treatment and recheck in 15 minutes. If there is no improvement, the patient should contact a physician.
	Sources of carbohydrates and suitable portions. There are three main sources of carbohydrates—milk, fruits, and starches (sugars and complex). Stress the importance of having some form of carbohydrate at every meal, especially complex carbohydrates to prevent hypoglycemia.
	Medications and insulin regimen.
	Timing of meals is extremely important with patients who administer insulin for blood glucose control. Rapid-acting insulin such as Lispro and Aspart should be administered when the patient sits down to eat. For patients with type 2 diabetes, there should be no carbohydrate loading at a meal because this puts stress on the already-compromised pancreas. Encourage patients not to skip meals; this could lead to hypoglycemia.
	Hemoglobin AIC. Hemoglobin AIC measures how controlled the blood glucose has been over a 3- to 6-month period. Goal is < 7% (Joslin Clinical Guidelines, 2006).
	Blood pressure. Blood pressure is the force blood exerts against the arterial walls as it is pumped through the body by the heart. High blood pressure occurs when this force is too strong (Gordon, 2006). The blood pressure goal for people with diabetes is < 130/80 mmHg.
	Lipid profile. People with diabetes are at increased risk for coronary artery disease and should have their lipids checked often. Explain "good" cholesterol (HDL), "bad" cholesterol (LDL), and total cholesterol and the acceptable values for each. Exercise helps to improve good cholesterol.
	See the section under hyperlipidemia for lipid goals.
	Sick days. If patient becomes sick with poor appetite, encourage regular juice, yogurt, soup, applesauce, and pudding with extra fluids. Monitor glucose every 2–4 hours.
	Continue medication/insulin as prescribed unless informed otherwise by the physician. If illness lasts longer than a day and is accompanied by fever, nausea/vomiting, or uncontrolled blood sugar, contact the physician immediately.

(continues)

Medical Condition	What to Teach
Diabetes (continued)	**Exercise.** Exercise helps to lower blood sugar, which can create the need to modify medication for blood glucose control. With any strenuous activity, patients should check blood sugar before, during, and after activity. If blood sugar is < 100 mg/dL, the patient should ingest 15–30 grams of carbohydrates (CHO). In type 1 diabetes, if fasting blood sugar is > 250 mg/dL with the presence of ketosis, avoid exercise. It is recommended that 15 grams of carbohydrate be given for 30–60 minutes of activity. Hydration is important before and during exercise to prevent hyperglycemia. Patients should always carry some form of CHO, including glucose tablets, as well as identification. They should avoid exercise in extreme weather.

Alcohol consumption. Alcohol can cause a drop in blood sugar and therefore should be consumed with meals. Alcohol, however, is contraindicated with some antihypertensive medications and should be avoided. Women should have no more than one drink a day and men no more than two drinks a day.

A drink is considered:

• A 5-oz glass of wine

• 1 ½ oz distilled spirits (e.g., vodka, gin, whiskey)

• 12 oz beer

Diabetic ketoacidosis (DKA). Diabetic ketoacidosis occurs more frequently in type 1 diabetes in which the blood sugar level is significantly increased due to inadequate insulin. Fat is therefore used for energy and ketones are formed. Ketones are poisonous and, if untreated, can lead to coma and death. Symptoms of DKA include fruity odor, increased thirst, urination, loss of appetite, labored breathing, fatigue, and dehydration. Patient should check for ketones in the urine when blood glucose is > 240 mg/dL, especially on sick days. The diagnostic criteria for DKA are blood glucose over 250 mg/dL, arterial pH below 7.3, bicarbonate concentration below 15 mEq/L, and moderate ketonuria or ketonemia (Kitabchi, et al., 2001). |
| **Gestational Diabetes** | **Complications of gestational diabetes**. If blood sugar is uncontrolled, there is an increased risk of hypoglycemia, difficulty during delivery due to size of the baby, with the risk of clavicle fracture. Stillbirth is also a possibility.

Glucose monitoring with acceptable goals.

Check blood sugar right after waking up. Blood sugar goals:

• Before breakfast 80–120 mg/dL

• 1 hour after meals <140 mg/dL

• 2 hours after meals ≤ 120 mg/dL

Meal planning. No juice, fruit, or other simple carbohydrates at breakfast. Breakfast may consist of complex carbohydrates and a protein item. Strive for three small meals with snacks in between meals. Include protein and fat at each meal to reduce hyperglycemia. |

Medical Condition	What to Teach
Inflammatory Bowel Disease (IBD)	The two most common forms of IBD are Crohn's disease and ulcerative colitis, which occurs with chronic inflammation of the gastrointestinal (GI) tract.

Diet. Calories and protein should be high to prevent malnutrition and weight loss. Limit dairy products. Choose lactose-free products. Patients may have cheese and yogurt.

Patients should follow these recommendations:

Avoid high-fat foods; follow a low-fat diet. Consider medium-chain triglycerides in the presence of steatorrhea.

Follow a low-fiber diet in the initial "flare-up" of the disease, and then increase fiber gradually, primarily soluble fiber, such as oats. Avoid raw fruits and vegetables. Adequate fluid intake is necessary as fiber is increased.

Recommend small, frequent meals and discourage use of alcohol, carbonated beverages, and caffeine-containing products because these increase intestinal activity.

Include iron-rich foods—meat, chicken, dark green leafy vegetables.

Dietary supplementation. With the loss of blood due to bloody diarrhea, iron, folic acid, and vitamin B_{12} may be necessary to treat anemia. Other supplements include calcium and vitamin D to prevent osteoporosis. |
| **End-Stage Liver Disease (ESLD)** | **Explain what happens when the liver is damaged.** The liver converts food into nutrients and stores vitamins, minerals, and sugar. It helps the body to get rid of toxic substances that can harm the body. When the liver is damaged, these functions are impaired.

Complications of ESLD.

Hepatic Encephalopathy

Patients may experience personality changes, mild confusion, impaired coordination, speech problems, loss of consciousness, coma, and possibly death. This results from a buildup of ammonia, which is toxic to the brain.

Portal Hypertension

This is an elevated blood pressure in the portal vein that carries nutrients from the GI tract to the liver. This occurs due to an obstruction of blood flow to the liver.

Fat Malabsorption

This results in a deficiency in fat-soluble vitamins and contributes to undernourishment (Henkel & Buchman, 2006).

Esophageal Varices

This is a deadly complication of ESLD in which there is bleeding in the esophagus and stomach due to portal hypertension. |

(continues)

Medical Condition	What to Teach
End-Stage Liver Disease (ESLD) (continued)	*Ascites* This is a condition in which fluids accumulate in the peritoneal cavity and, if not treated, can affect respiratory and kidney functions. Fluid restriction may be necessary. **Diet.** Diet should be high in calories, carbohydrate, and protein of high biological value. Patients should limit sodium intake and avoid alcohol and drugs. Reduce fat intake if steatorrhea is present. **Medication and supplementation.** Lactulose and/or neomycin are usually given to reduce ammonia levels. These may cause diarrhea but should be taken as prescribed. The physician may recommend niacin, thiamine, folate, vitamin B_6, zinc, and magnesium as nutritional supplements, especially for the patient with a history of alcoholism. Diuretics may be prescribed for fluid retention.
Short Bowel Syndrome (on oral nutrition)	**Complications associated with Short Bowel Syndrome.** The patient may experience chronic diarrhea resulting in loss of electrolytes and possible dehydration as well as deficiency in important nutrients due to malabsorption. **Diet.** Diet should be high in protein and complex carbohydrates. Patients should avoid high-fat foods. Small, frequent meals are recommended. Encourage the patient to limit sweets due to rapid gastric emptying following bowel resection. If diarrhea is exacerbated with the use of milk, advise the patient to have lactose-free milk and/or yogurt and cheese. Include banana for potassium and to aid diarrhea. Boiled rice, applesauce, and yogurt can also relieve diarrhea. Fluid intake should be adequate to prevent dehydration and should contain sodium and glucose. No "plain" water should be used. Oral rehydration solution (ORS) is recommended (Buchman, 2004). Restrict caffeine and alcohol. If the colon is intact, patient should follow an oxalate-restricted diet to reduce the risk of developing calcium-oxalate kidney stones. Foods high in oxalate include tea, cola drinks, chocolate, nuts, green leafy vegetables, celery, strawberries, blueberries, and tangerines (Bernard & Shaw, 1993). Emphasize intake of iron-rich foods. **Dietary supplementation.** Vitamins, especially B_{12}, folate, and other water-soluble vitamins, are needed to prevent nutrient deficiency and to treat megaloblastic anemia. Calcium supplement and vitamins A, D, and K may also be prescribed.
Diverticulosis	**Explain diverticulosis.** The formation of bulging pouches along the walls of the colon that may be caused by a history of low dietary fiber. **High-fiber diet.** Sources of fiber are fruits, vegetables, bran, oatmeal, legumes, and whole grains.

Medical Condition	What to Teach
Diverticulosis (continued)	**How to incorporate fiber in the diet.** Recommend patients increase fiber gradually to prevent bloating and gas. They can add fruits to cereal, add All Bran to farina. They can use oatmeal instead of flour as a binder for meatballs/meatloaf, use recipes containing peas/beans, use fresh as well as dried fruits as snacks. They can switch to brown rice and whole wheat bread, include moderate servings of vegetables at lunch and dinner, and use whole wheat flour instead of white flour.
	Fluids. As fiber is increased, fluid intake must also be increased. At least eight glasses of fluids are recommended to prevent constipation.
	Explain diverticulitis.
	Diverticulitis occurs when the bulging pouches (diverticula) along the walls of the colon become inflamed and infected. Symptoms may include rectal bleeding, resulting in possible anemia and low albumin levels. Patients may also experience constipation and diarrhea.
	Dietary treatment. Patients should follow a low-residue diet during the flare-up of diveriticulitis and, once resolved, increase fiber gradually. They should increase fluid intake. It may be necessary to follow a low-fat diet.
	Low-Residue Diet
	Avoid raw vegetables and vegetables with seeds, cereal, bread, or crackers containing whole grains, nuts, or seeds.
	Avoid dried fruits and fruits with skin, peas, beans, and potatoes with skin.
	Patients may have cooked vegetables without seeds and skin, strained vegetable juice, canned or cooked fruits, applesauce, ripe bananas, white rice, potatoes without skins, farina, and grits.
	Increase Protein
	Include tender cooked chicken, fish and other seafoods, beef, liver, and pork. Include dairy products—milk, eggs, and cheese.
	Increase Fluid Intake
	Include 6–8 cups of fluids/day.
Colostomy/ Ileostomy	**Explain rationale for low-residue diet.** To promote healing of the bowel after surgery. This might take 6–8 weeks (see low-residue diet earlier).
	Progression to a regular/high-fiber diet. Patients should add one high-fiber food at a time and chew properly.
	Increase fluid intake to prevent constipation.
	Limit foods that may produce excessive gas, for example, asparagus, cabbage, broccoli, beer or carbonated beverages, onions, egg, and fish. These foods can also produce an odor.

(continues)

Medical Condition	What to Teach
Colostomy/ Ileostomy (continued)	If diarrhea occurs, use Gatorade or other electrolyte-containing fluids instead of water to replace sodium and potassium. Limit fiber and include banana, applesauce, boiled rice, and yogurt to alleviate diarrhea.
	Food blockage. It is important that patients chew food thoroughly to prevent food blockage, which can lead to dehydration. Symptoms of food blockage are as follows:
	• Thin liquid discharge
	• Increased volume output
	• Strong unpleasant odor
	• Cramping
	• Distended abdomen
	• Vomiting
	• No output
	Patients should contact a physician if blockage continues for more than 4 hours.
Gastric Bypass Surgery	**Nutritional complications associated with surgery:**
	• Nausea and vomiting.
	• Bloating.
	• Dumping syndrome characterized by feelings of fullness, stomach cramping, diarrhea, weakness, sweating, and fast heart rate. Dumping syndrome occurs when food passes too quickly from the stomach to the small intestine.
	• Deficiency of important vitamins and minerals. Will need to take vitamins and mineral supplements for life.
	Diet progression.
	Explain what constitutes
	• Clear liquid diet
	• Full liquid diet
	• Pureed diet
	• Regular diet
	Fluids, preferably water, should be about 64 oz per day.
	Patients should choose low-fat foods and increase protein-rich foods. They should eat slowly and chew foods thoroughly.
	How to reduce/treat dumping syndrome:
	• Drink liquids 30–45 minutes after meals.
	• Consume small, frequent meals.
	• Avoid simple sugars.
	• Decrease intake of lactose-containing products.
	• When full, stop eating.

Medical Condition	What to Teach
Home Enteral Nutrition	**The formula.** Explain the nutritional content of the formula, its purpose, and administration. Be specific about the amount and frequency of the formula. It is helpful to give the patient a specific schedule to follow. Unopened and partially used formula must be stored at the temperature recommended by the manufacturer. Products should be inspected for contents and expiration date (American Society for Parenteral and Enteral Nutrition Board of Directors and the Standards for Specialized Nutrition Support Task Force et al., 2005).
	Discuss appropriate hang time for formula with the patient.
	Provide information to or refer the patient to community resources that can replenish the supply of formula. The social worker is a good resource person for more information on obtaining enteral nutrition formulas and supplies.
	Water flushes. Explain the purpose of water flushes—to clear the tube and provide adequate hydration. Give specific instructions regarding water flushes before, after, and in between feedings. Caution patient to adhere to specified water flushes to reduce the risk of overhydration.
	Sanitation. Advise patients to wash hands properly before administering feed and wash top of cans of formula before opening to reduce the risk of infection. Supplies used for administering formula should be properly sanitized. They should discard leftover formula.
	Positioning. Patients should always maintain a close to 90° angle for feeding and remain in a seated position for at least half an hour before lying down to prevent regurgitation of formula.
	Complications associated with tube feeding. Diarrhea, constipation, abdominal discomfort, nausea, vomiting, aspiration, dehydration, and overhydration are some complications the patient might experience while on tube feeding. Inform patients of the signs and symptoms of these complications.
	Advise the patient to contact a physician should these problems develop.
	Regular bloodwork is important to ensure that there are no metabolic issues.

(continues)

Medical Condition	What to Teach
Home Parenteral Nutrition	**Complications associated with parenteral nutrition:** • Increased risk of infection • Fluid imbalances that can lead to hyperglycemia and dehydration • Electrolyte imbalances, especially potassium and sodium **Home care:** • Keep the solution refrigerated. • Remove the solution from the refrigerator and allow it to reach room temperature prior to infusion. • Report any signs of redness, swelling, or drainage at the catheter site. • Report foul-smelling or limited output of urine. • Follow discharge instructions given by the nurse/physician. • Keep follow-up appointments for bloodwork. • Monitor weight daily and report any significant loss/gain.

SUMMARY

It is not unusual to discover after a teaching session that some important information was not covered in the session. This chapter provides you with information on various aspects of the medical condition affecting the patient. Although it may not be feasible to cover all areas outlined here at one time, you must select, based on the number of sessions you have with the patient, the areas that need immediate attention.

REVIEW QUESTIONS

1. You receive a medical consult for a patient with gestational diabetes. Develop a meal plan for this patient. What will be your education focus and why?
2. Patient X is being discharged home on enteral nutrition formula. You have been asked to do diet teaching before he leaves the hospital. What important information would you cover in your presentation?

REFERENCES

American Diabetes Association. (2009). Diabetes care. Retrieved September 17, 2009, from http://care.diabetesjournals.org/content/32/Supplement_1

American Society for Parenteral and Enteral Nutrition Board of Directors and the Standards for Specialized Nutrition Support Task Force et al. (2005). Standards for specialized nutrition support: Home care patients. *Nutrition in Clinical Practice, 20*(5), 579.

Bartlett J., & Gallant J. (2005–2006). *Medical management of HIV infection.* Baltimore: Johns Hopkins University School of Medicine.

Bernard, D. K., & Shaw, M. J. (1993). Principles of nutrition therapy for short bowel syndrome. *Nutrition in Clinical Practice, 8*(4), 153–162.

Buchman, A. L., & Henkel, S. A. (2006). Nutritional support in chronic liver disease. *National Clininical Practice Gastroenterology and Hepatology, 3*(4), 202–209.

Buchman, A. (2004). The medical and surgical management of short bowel syndrome. *Medscape General Medicine, 6*(2), 12.

Food Marketing Institute. (1996, March). *The food keeper: A consumer guide to food quality and safe handling.* Arlington, VA: Author.

Gordon, M. (2006). *Manual of nursing diagnosis* (11th ed.). Sudbury, MA: Jones and Bartlett.

Joslin Diabetes Center. (n.d.). *Joslin clinical guidelines.* Retrieved October 1, 2009, from http://www.joslin.org/managing_your_diabetes_joslin_clinical_guidelines.asp

Kitabchi, A. E., Umpierrez, G. E., Murphy, M., Barrett, E. J., Kreisberg, R. A., & Malone, J. I., et al. (2001). Hyperglycemia crises in patients with diabetes mellitus. *Diabetes Care, American Diabetes Association, 24*(suppl), 583–590.

McVan, L., & Cahill, M. (1987). *Patient teaching (Nurses Reference Library).* North Wales, PA: Springhouse Publishing Co.

ADDITIONAL RESOURCES

The National Kidney Foundation: http://www.kidney.org

Documentation

CHAPTER 9

The Legal Aspects of Documentation

WHY DOCUMENT?

Documentation serves to meet the needs of the patients and also plays an important role in the facility's ability to maintain Joint Commission accreditation and qualify for financial reimbursement from Medicare, Medicaid, and other third-party payers. Documentation also serves to protect you in your practice. Always document with the law in mind because you never know when you will be asked to defend what you wrote.

THE PURPOSE OF DOCUMENTATION

The purpose of documentation is to create a complete picture of the patient for whom services are provided. It provides guidance to the physician and other members of the healthcare team regarding appropriate medications and treatments based on the patient's physical and mental status. Documentation must always address the need for intervention, adjustment to plan if any, and the patient's response to the intervention. There should always be justification for the continuation or discontinuation of the plan of care.

Documentation helps you develop an appropriate plan of care for the patient. It helps to coordinate care effort and techniques among all disciplines because proper documentation provides needed information for all disciplines. Communication between clinicians and everyone who documents in the patient's chart is extremely important to ensure continuity of care and help prevent ambiguity. Attending care plan meetings and being involved in grand tours create cohesiveness on the healthcare team.

Documentation provides the means with which you can monitor and evaluate quality of care and it also serves as a research and continuing education tool.

THE MEDICAL RECORD AS A LEGAL DOCUMENT

The medical record is a legal document. It protects clinicians and the facility and therefore should be clear and precise, without ambiguity. The medial record holds the memory of all disciplines associated with the patient. It provides proof of the care that the resident/patient has received during the time he or she was admitted to the facility.

In the event of a lawsuit, your documentation can defend you if it is properly done. A lawsuit can be filed several years after you have documented on a patient, so the medical record serves as your memory. Judges rely heavily on documentation concerning behaviors and resident reactions to situations. Accurate documentation assists lawyers and judges in making appropriate decisions. "While traditionally, medical malpractice suits have targeted physicians, trend data suggest an increasing number of RDs (registered dietitians), particularly those in clinical care, are being named in practice-related lawsuits" (Moores, 2007).

COMMON DOCUMENTATION ISSUES IN MALPRACTICE LAWSUITS

By Nancy Collins, PhD, RD, LDN. Originally appeared in the October 2007 issue of *ECPN* magazine for extended care professionals.

1. **Height and Weight Inaccuracies**
   In some facilities, weight inconsistencies are so common in charts it has become quasi-acceptable to chart "weight appears erroneous."

2. **Improper Monitoring of Meal Intake**

    Most facilities have adopted a system of recording meal consumption on a flow sheet using terms such as excellent, good, fair, poor or refused meal. In a typical month, that equates to 90 entries, or 30 days with three meals per day. These sheets are not always completed properly. For example, if a box is not filled in, it can appear the resident did not receive a meal.

    In other instances, it is obvious the entire flow sheet was filled out at one time with the same pen, the same intake amounts every day and in the same handwriting. This known as "dry-labbing" and it is a form of cheating.

    Keep in mind time sheets are often subpoenaed and the initials of the employee on the flow sheet can easily be correlated with the days the employee was scheduled to work.

3. **Timeliness of Follow-up on Nutrition Recommendation**

    Lawyers argue delays may have harmed the patient, yet many facilities do not have standing protocols in place to deal with common issues such as unintended weight loss. Standing protocols would eliminate the need for some orders and shorten the time lapse in acting upon nutrition recommendation.

4. **Tube Feeding Intentions**

    If a patient continues to lose weight despite optimal nutrition interventions, it may indicate a disease reaching its end stage. In some cases, no further nutrition intervention is warranted. But few medical records contain clear documentation that this fact was communicated to family members and the patient. This lack of documentation can lead to the claim that the family desired a tube feeding that could have prevented a further weight decline.

5. **Inadequate Staffing**

    The issue of nutrition staffing often arises in litigation because many facilities do not employ staff dietitians but use consultants. And while certified dietary managers and dietetic technicians, registered, play an important role on the health-care team, they work under the supervision of a registered dietitian and are not trained to independently provide care to highly complicated patients. Another question that frequently arises: Could an RD adequately supervise the nutrition team members given the number of hours in her contract?

6. **Services Does Not Meet Expectations**

    Seemingly small complaints that do not cause medical harm to patients can cause harm to families' perception of the care the patient received. Family members often do not complain in depositions about the medical care; they complain about laundry, food, cleanliness of the facility and the way they were treated. And as experience has shown, testimony of these experiences can have an impact on the case.

7. **Nutritional Nonadherence**
   While many practitioners believe it is within a patient's right to refuse an unwanted dietary intervention, some facilities require patient to sign a paper stating they understand the consequences of their actions, particularly if the action could compromise the effectiveness of treatment while at the facility.

Source: © American Dietetic Association. All rights reserved. License # ADAT 4812

GENERAL INFORMATION REGARDING DOCUMENTATION

Following are some general guidelines to follow for effective documentation:

- Never remove a document from the medical record and replace it with a copy; this is illegal and is punishable by law.
- Don't chart ahead of time. It is considered fraud to chart that you did something that you did not actually do.
- Whatever care you offer the patient, document, document, document! *If it is not documented, it was never done.*
- Always provide supporting evidence for nutritional diagnoses, for example, "patient at high risk for aspiration secondary to tube feeding, decreased level of consciousness, increased gastric residual, vomiting episodes and delayed gastric emptying."
- Never alter a patient's record—this is illegal. If you must make changes, do an addendum. If you remember an important point after your documentation is done, chart the new information with a notation that it is a "late entry" or an addendum to a progress note. Include the date and time the late entry was written, and refer the reader to a previous note for other information (e.g., 8/01/07: 9 am Addendum to progress note 7/28/07); continue entry, and sign.
- Always chart noncompliance and refusal. A patient has a right to refuse treatment including therapeutic diet. Factors that influence refusal may include the patient's value system, health beliefs, cultural

influences, fear and anxiety, spiritual values, client–provider relationship, paranoia, or addiction.

Once the patient's ability to give informed consent is established, you should discuss with the patient or significant other(s) their understanding of the situation and the consequences of their choice to refuse treatment. If, after discussion, the patient insists on refusal, you must accept the patient's choice and document the conversation and outcome. Some facilities require the patient to sign a "refusal of treatment" form.

- Do not falsify the medical record. For example, if you are unable to obtain weight for an assessment, document "unable to obtain weight at this time [state the reason, for example, patient in physical therapy]. Will follow up with next visit."

- If, after writing your note, the physician does not agree with your recommendation, contact the physician for a reasonable answer for refusing the recommendation and, based on the outcome of the conversation, write an addendum to the note. The following is an example: "After discussion with MD, it was felt that prognosis for patient CH is poor and that he would not benefit from tube feeding at this time. Will continue IVF and follow up progress."

  An alternative to the preceding situation is for the physician to write, "Nutrition consult appreciated, but due to poor prognosis recommendation will not be followed at this time."

- If the diet the physician orders is deemed incorrect for the patient's diagnosis, contact the physician and provide supporting evidence for the correct diet and have the MD discontinue the previous order and write a new order for the correct diet.

- Do not use your documentation to place blame on someone else or another department. It is important to maintain a professional attitude at all times and be mindful of the fact that every member of the healthcare team works together for the optimum care of the patient.

- If the patient's caloric intake is less than the calculated requirement, as in the case of some patients on tube feeding, your note should reflect justification for the reduced caloric intake.

- Avoid the following phrases/words when documenting in the patient's record because they provide little or no information: "doing well," "appears healthy," "nice," "good day."

- If you are brought up on trial for misconduct, get a lawyer. It is advisable to have your own professional liability insurance even if your employer has a policy, because lawsuits can run into the thousands of dollars.
- Adhering to company policy helps to protect you in the event of a lawsuit. Be familiar with the standards of your company and do not deviate from them to satisfy a disgruntled patient/resident. Document any conflict you may encounter while implementing the company policy and bring it to the attention of your superior(s).

MECHANICS OF GOOD DOCUMENTATION

Here are some recommendations for creating useful documentation:

- *Always write legibly.* Remember, you are not the only one reading the patient's chart, and each discipline's documentation is important to provide optimum care to the patient.
- *Always include patient identification on all forms.* Make sure the chart matches the person you are documenting on. If you document in the wrong chart, draw a line through the documentation, write, "wrong pt," and initial it.
- *Date and time all notes.* This is extremely important should a legal matter arise regarding patient care. Do not back-date notes. Always date the note the day and time it was written.
- *Notes should be factual.* Leave out opinions except when they are related to recommendations for the nutritional care of the patient. Do not fabricate information.
- *Write what you see, hear, feel, or smell* (American Dietetic Association, 2009). Document the patient's report as given. If a patient curses during an interview, write exactly what he said because such an outburst may warrant the need for psychological evaluation. Do not paraphrase or write what you think the patient meant. You can describe the patient's behavior, but avoid using derogatory remarks or adjectives to describe the patient.
- *Always write in ink, blue or black, depending on the policy of your facility.*

- *Always complete the assessment form in its entirety.* Do not leave blanks on any form. If a section is not applicable, write N/A in the blank.
- *Sign all notes with your appropriate credentials/title.*
- *Avoid jargon and inappropriate abbreviations.* Use only abbreviations that are accepted by your facility.
- *Never use correction fluid or tape in the medical record.* This suggests that you are covering up something. If you make an error, strike through with one line, initial and date, and then continue your note. If you need to add or make changes to a note you have written, write an addendum using the current date. You may include a line referring the reader to a previous note. This same principle applies to making late entries in the chart.
- *Always paint a complete picture of the situation.* Clinical description must be precise and detailed, leaving no room for ambiguity. If a nutrition-related diagnosis or biochemical data are not addressed, it might constitute negligence on your part, especially if complications develop as a result of not addressing the issue.
- *Make sure your notes correspond with your care plan.* Always update care plans with new information.
- *Always document and follow up what is told to you by other disciplines regarding the care of the patient.* For example, the nurse might report, patient is vomiting, is constipated, has poor oral intake. It is advisable to have the informant document the problem in the chart, before doing your assessment. If this is not done, your note might read, "per nursing, patient CH vomited about 200 cc of undigested food following evening meal," and then continue with your assessment.
- *Never skip lines in the progress notes.* If your documentation ends in the middle of a line, draw a line through the blank space and sign your name with title at the end of the line.
- *Check spelling for accuracy.* It is always helpful to have a medical dictionary on hand for spelling checking.
- *Document with the law in mind.* You never know who will be reading your notes. Leave no loophole that will open you up to an investigation. You must be able to defend in court what you have written.
- *Read the notes of other clinicians so that there is no conflict in the documentation.* For example, the nurse's notes read, "Pt noted with B/L

edema," but your assessment says, "No edema." Conflict in documentation can be a loophole for an investigation.

- Should there be a conflict in the documentation, be quick to point this out to the writer of the note that so it can be addressed immediately.
- *Never a chart a problem without documenting what you are doing about it.*

     For example: **Problem**: Pt refuses Ensure supplement for weight gain.

     Plan: Will offer milkshake, ice cream, and continue to monitor oral intake and weight.

- *Encourage others to document relevant information that they share with you.*
- *Always chart what you report to other healthcare providers.*

DOCUMENTATION USING THE NUTRITION CARE PROCESS

The American Dietetic Association has adopted the following format for documentation used in collaboration with the Nutrition Care Process and model. Details of each step are covered in more detail in various chapters of this book.

A: Assessment, where information on the patient is obtained from the chart review and patient/family interview. This includes anthropometrics, diet and medical history, biochemical data, and psychosocial data.

D: Diagnosis, where the nutrition problem is identified with supporting evidence. A clear, concise statement of nutrition diagnosis(es) is written in the general format: "Diagnosis" related to "etiology" as evidenced by "signs and symptoms."

   Example: "Weight loss related to chewing difficulty with meal refusal, evidenced by 10-pound weight loss in 30 days." If the patient presents with no nutrition problem that warrants nutrition intervention, the words "no nutrition diagnosis at this time" may be documented in the medical record.

I: Intervention, to address the nutrition problem or diagnosis. Intervention may include diet prescription, recommendation, and implementation. Goals are developed, and the patient is involved in the goal-setting process. Education and counseling are documented in this section.

M: Monitoring of progress to see whether goals/objectives are met. Monitoring procedures may include regular weight checks, review of biochemical data, compliance with diet recommendations, dietary intake records, tolerance of diet, nutritional supplementation, and tube feeding.

E: Evaluate the monitoring procedures. This section measures outcomes relevant to the nutrition diagnosis and intervention plans and goals. It compares current findings with previous status or reference standards and determines factors that help or hinder progress.

Documentation using the Nutrition Care Process ensures that the cause of the nutrition problems is identified and intervention including goals/objectives and education is in place to address/correct the problem(s). Follow-up through monitoring and evaluation allows you to identify barriers to achieving goals and also to modify current goals for compliance and positive outcome.

SUMMARY

Proper documentation can defend the writer in the event of a lawsuit. It is considered negligence if a nutrition-related problem is identified and not addressed. Communication with other members of the healthcare team provides more information on the patient. It is important to adhere to facilities' guidelines when documenting in the medical record because failure to do so could result in you having no company support in the case of a lawsuit.

REVIEW QUESTIONS

1. You recommend a diet change for a patient, but the physician disagrees with your recommendation. What would you do?
2. You requested weight on Patient S on several occasions, but it is still not available. You are unable to complete your nutrition assessment because there is no weight for the patient. How would you handle this situation, and what would you document in the medical record?

3. Patient JB was referred to you for nutrition counseling following admission to the AIDS unit at your hospital. He is a 45-year-old man, with a height of 5 feet 9 inches, and he weighs 130 pounds. He is diagnosed with AIDS and has reported nausea, loss of appetite, and persistent diarrhea. Three months ago, he weighed 160 pounds. Albumin is 2.8 mg/dL. Using the format of the Nutrition Care Process, prepare a plan of care for this patient.

REFERENCES

American Dietetic Association. (2008a). Nutrition Care Process and Model Part I: The 2008 update. *Journal of the American Dietetic Association, 108*(7), 1113–1117.

American Dietetic Association. (2008b). Nutrition Care Process part II: Using the International Dietetics and Nutrition terminology to document the Nutrition Care Process. *Journal of the American Dietetic Association, 108*(8), 1287–1293.

American Dietetic Association. (2009). *Medical nutrition therapy documentation.* Retrieved October 5, 2009, from http://eatright.org/cps/rde/xchg/ada/hs.xsl/nutrition_12896_ENU_HTML.htm

Gialanella, K. (2004, June). *Documentation.* Retrieved October 7, 2009, from http://lpn.advanceweb.com/Article/Documentation.aspx

Moores, S. (2007). Risky business: Protecting yourself in a litigious world. *ADA Times, 5*(2), 12–17.

Appendix

APPROVED ABBREVIATION LIST FOR SOME COMMON DIAGNOSES AND TERMS

AA	Alcoholics Anonymous
AAA	abdominal aortic aneurysm
abd	abdomen
ABE	acute bacterial endocarditis
ABGs	arterial blood gases
abn	abnormal
ABP	arterial blood pressure
ABR	auditory brainstem response
ABS	acute brain syndrome
ACTD	actinomycin-D
ACTH	adrenocorticotropic hormone
ACS	acute coronary syndrome
ACVD	acute cardiovascular disease
ad lib	as much as needed
ADLs	activities of daily living
A. fib	atrial fibrillation
A. flutter	atrial flutter
AFB	acid fast bacillus
AFO	ankle foot orthosis
AGA	appropriate for gestational age
AGN	acute glomerulonephritis
AKA	above-the-knee amputation
ALL	acute lymphocytic leukemia

AMA	against medical advice
AMI	acute myocardial infarction
ANA	antinuclear antibodies
ANF	antinuclear factor
AOB	alcohol on breath
ARF	acute renal failure
ASA	aspirin
ASHD	arteriosclerotic cardiovascular disease
ATN	acute tubular necrosis
B	bilateral
Ba	barium
BG	blood glucose
BKA	below-knee amputation
BLS	basic life support
bm	bowel movement
BMI	body mass index
BMR	basal metabolic rate
BP	blood pressure
BPD	bronchopulmonary dysplasia
BPH	benign prostatic hypertrophy
bpm	beats per minute
BUN	blood urea nitrogen
Ca	calcium
CA	carcinoma
CABG	coronary artery bypass graft
CAD	coronary artery disease
CAH	chronic active hepatitis
CAPD	chronic ambulatory peritoneal dialysis
cath	catheter
CBC	complete blood count
CBI	continuous bladder irrigation
CHB	complete heart block
CHD	congenital heart disease, coronary heart disease
Chemo	chemotherapy
CHF	congestive heart failure
CIS	carcinoma in situ

CKD	chronic kidney disease
CNS	central nervous system
c/o	complains of
COPD	chronic obstructive pulmonary disease
CPA	cerebellopontine angle
CPAP	continuous positive airway pressure
CPH	chronic persistent hepatitis
CPR	cardiopulmonary resuscitation
CRF	chronic renal failure
CRIF	closed reduction internal fixation
C/S	cesarean section
CSF	cerebrospinal fluid
CSOM	chronic serous otitis media
CT	computerized tomography
CTS	carpal tunnel syndrome
ctx	contractions
CVA	cerebovascular accident
CVP	central venous pressure
CXR	chest X-ray
cysto	cystoscopy
D&C	dilation and curettage
DBP	diastolic blood pressure
decub	decubitus
DEXA	dual energy X-ray absorptiometry
D5S	5% dextrose in saline
D5W	5% dextrose in water
DFA	difficulty falling asleep
DI	diabetes insipidus
DJD	degenerative joint disease
DM	diabetes mellitus
DMARD	disease-modifying antirheumatic drug
DNA	deoxyribonucleic acid
D/NS	dextrose in normal saline
DOA	dead on arrival
DOE	dyspnea on exertion
DRE	digital rectal examination
DSD	dry, sterile dressing

DTR	deep tendon reflexes
DUB	dysfunctional uterine bleeding
DUI	driving under the influence
DVT	deep vein thrombosis
D/W	dextrose in water
DWI	driving while intoxicated
Dx	diagnosis
E. coli	*Escherichia coli*
EBL	estimated blood loss
EC	enteric-coated
ECF	extracellular fluid
ECG/EKG	electrocardiogram
Echo	echocardiogram
ECT	electroconvulsive therapy
ED	erectile dysfunction
EEG	electroencephalogram
EENT	eye, ear, nose, and throat
EGD	esophagogastroduodenoscopy
elix	elixir
EM	electron microscopy
EMG	electromyography
ENT	ear, nose, throat
eos	eosinophils
ER	extended release
ESR	erythrocyte sedimentation rate
ESRD	end-stage renal disease
ETOH	ethyl alcohol
ETT	endotracheal tube
exc	excision
exp	expired
F	Fahrenheit, fluoride
FBS	fasting blood sugar
FEV	forced expiratory volume
FFP	fresh frozen plasma
FOB	fecal occult blood
FS	fingerstick

FSH	follicle-stimulating hormone
F/U	follow-up
FUO	fever of unknown origin
FVC	forced vital capacity
fx	fracture
GERD	gastroesophageal reflux disease
GFR	glomerular filtration rate
GGT	gamma-glutamyl transferase
GGTP	gamma-glutamyl transpeptidase
GH	growth hormone
Gi, Gl	gastrointestinal
GP	glycoprotein
GSW	gunshot wounds
Gtt	a drop, drops
GU	genitourinary
HA, HAL	hyperalimentation
HbA1c	glycosylated hemoglobin
HBV	hepatitis B virus
HCG, hCG	human chorionic gonadotropin
HCM	hypercalcemia of malignancy
HCT	hematocrit
HCV	hepatitis C virus
HDL	high-density lipoprotein
Hg	mercury
H&H	hematocrit and hemoglobin
HIT	Heparin-induced thrombocytopenia
HOB	head of bed
HR	heart rate
HRT	hormone replacement therapy
HSE	herpes simplex encephalitis
HSV	herpes simplex virus
Ht	height
HTN	hypertension
IA	intra-arterial
IBD	inflammatory bowel disease

IBS	irritable bowel syndrome
IBW	ideal body weight
ICP	intracranial pressure
ICU	intensive care unit
Im, IM	intramuscular
Inh	inhalation
INR	international normalized ratio
I&O	intake and output
IOP	intraocular pressure
IPPB	intermittent positive pressure breathing
Iv, IV	intravenous
JT	jejunostomy tube
JTF	jejunostomy tube feeding
JVD	jugular venous distention
K	potassium
KCL	potassium chloride
Kg	kilogram (2.2 lb)
Kj	knee jerk
KVO	keep vein open
LBP	low back pain
LDH	lactic dehydrogenase
LDL	low density lipoprotein
LFTs	liver function tests
LHRH	luteinizing hormone-releasing hormone
LLE	left lower extremity
LMP	last menstrual period
LOC	level of consciousness/loss of consciousness
LTG	long term goal
LV	left ventricular
LVE	left ventricular end diastolic
LVEF	left ventricular ejection fraction
LVH	left ventricular hypertrophy
MAC	*Mycobacterium avium* complex
MAOI	monoamine oxidase inhibitor

MAP	mean arterial pressure
MAR	medication administration record
MCH	mean corpuscular hemoglobin
MCV	mean corpuscular volume
MDRSP	multidrug-resistant *Streptococcus pneumoniae*
MI	myocardial infarction
MM	multiple myeloma
MME	Mini Mental Examination
MMSE	Mini Mental State (Status) Examination
MOM	milk of magnesia
MRI	magnetic resonance imaging
MS	multiple sclerosis
MTX	methotrexate
MU	million units
MVA	motor vehicle accident
NaCl	sodium chloride
NAD	no acute distress
NAS	no added salt
N/C	no complaints
NG	nasogastric
NGT	nasogastric tube
NKA	no known allergies
NKDA	no known drug allergies
NMS	neuroleptic malignant syndrome
NSAID	nonsteroidal anti-inflammatory drug
NSS	normal saline solution
NTG	nitroglycerin
NWB	non weight bearing
N&V	nausea and vomiting
O	oxygen
OC	oral contraceptive
OCD	obsessive-compulsive disorder
O.D.	right eye
OOB	out of bed
OR	operating room
O.S.	left eye

OT	occupational therapy
OTC	over the counter
O.U.	both eyes
PA	pulmonary artery
PAC	premature atrial contraction
PAF	paroxysmal atrial fibrillation or flutter
p.c.	after meals
PCA	patient-controlled analgesia
PCI	percutaneous coronary intervention
PCN	penicillin
PCP	*Pneumocystis carinii* pneumonia
PCWP	pulmonary capillary wedge pressure
PFTs	pulmonary function tests
Ph	hydrogen ion concentration
PID	pelvic inflammatory disease
PMH	past medical history
PND	paroxysmal nocturnal dyspnea
PO	by mouth
PR	by rectum
PRN	when needed or necessary
PSA	prostate-specific antigen
PT	prothrombin time, or physical therapy
PTA	prior to admission
PTCA	percutaneous transluminal coronary angioplasty
PTH	parathyroid hormone
PTSD	post-traumatic stress disorder
PTT	partial thromboplastin time
PUD	peptic ulcer disease
PVD	peripheral vascular disease
PVR	peripheral vascular resistance
RA	right atrium, or rheumatoid arthritis
RBC	red blood cell
RDA	Recommended Daily Allowance
REM	rapid eye movement
RICE	rest, ice, compression, and elevation
RNA	ribonucleic acid

R/O	rule out
ROM	range of motion
ROS	review of systems
RRMS	relapsing-remitting multiple sclerosis
R/T	related to
RTC	round the clock
RUQ	right upper quadrant
RV	right ventricular
Rx	symbol for prescription
SAH	subarachnoid hemorrhage
SARS	severe acute respiratory syndrome
SBP	systolic blood pressure
Sc, SC	subcutaneous
SCI	spinal cord injury
SCID	severe combined immunodeficiency disease
SGGT	serum gamma-glutamyl transpeptidase
SGOT	serum glutamic-oxaloacetic transaminase
SGPT	serum glumatic-pyruvic transaminase
SIADH	syndrome inappropriate antidiuretic hormone
SL	sublingual
SLE	system lupus erythematosus
SOB	shortness of breath
SSE	soap suds enema
SSNRI	selective serotonin norepinephrine reuptake inhibitor
SSRI	selective serotonin reuptake inhibitor
SSS	sick sinus syndrome
S&S	signs and symptoms
Stat	immediately
STD	sexually transmitted disease
STG	short-term goal
SV	stroke volume
SVT	supraventricular tachycardia
TB	tuberculosis
TCA	tricyclic antidepressant
TG	triglycerides
THR	total hip replacement

TIA	transient ischemic attack
TIBC	total iron binding capacity
TKR	total knee replacement
TNF	tumor necrosis factor
TPN	total parenteral nutrition
TSH	thyroid stimulating hormone
U/A	urinalysis
UGI	upper gastrointestinal
UO	urine output
URTI	upper respiratory tract infection
US	ultrasound
UTI	urinary tract infection
UV	ultraviolet
VA	visual acuity
VAD	venous access device
VF	ventricular fibrillation
VLDL	very low density lipoprotein
V.O	verbal order
VS	vital signs
VT	ventricular tachycardia
WBC	white blood cell
WF	white female
WM	white male
WNL	within normal limits
Wt	weight
XRT	radiation therapy

SYMBOLS

<	less than
>	greater than
°	degree
/	per
△	change
2°	secondary to
24°	24 hours
c̄	with
s̄	without
p̄	following
ā	preceding or before
↑	increase, increased, or higher
↓	decrease, decreased, or lower
♀	female
♂	male

Index

Figures and tables are indicated with *f* and *t* following the page number.

Abbreviation list for diagnoses and terminology, 181–190
Abilify (aripiprazole), 34
ACE (angiotensin-converting enzyme) inhibitors, 31
Activities of daily living (ADLs), 28
Acute malnutrition. *See* Malnutrition
Adjusted body weight determination, 13–14
Adolescents, 119–123, 126, 126*t*. *See also* Pediatric assessment
Adverse food reactions, 74. *See also* Food allergies and intolerance
AIDS. *See* HIV/AIDS
ALA (alpha-lipoic acid), 72–73
Albumin, 44*t*
Alcohol
    breastfeeding and, 104
    constipation caused by, 21
    fetal growth retardation and, 99
    hepatitis and, 37
    during pregnancy, 93
    triglyceride increase caused by, 29
Aldactone, 31, 32
Alpha-lipoic acid (ALA), 72–73
Alpha thalassemia, 64
Alzheimer's disease, 34
Amenorrhea, 122
American Dietetic Association, 3, 69. *See also* Nutrition Care Process

Amino acids, 36
Ammonia, 45*t*
Amputations, 8
Anabolism, 90
Analgesics, 50*t*
Android obesity, 86
Anemia, 40, 42
Angina, 29–30
Angiotensin-converting enzyme (ACE) inhibitors, 31
Angiotensin II receptor blockers (ARBs), 31
Anorexia nervosa, 18, 119–120
Antacids, 50*t*
Antianemics, 50*t*
Antibiotics, 39, 50*t*
Anticoagulants, 50*t*
Anticonvulsants, 40, 50*t*
Antidepressants, 33, 50*t*
Antidiarrheals, 50*t*
Antiemetics, 51*t*
Anti-GERD/proton pump inhibitors, 51*t*
Antigouts, 51*t*
Antihistamines, 52*t*
Antihyperlipidemics, 51*t*
Antihypertensives, 51*t*
Antimanics, 51*t*
Antineoplastics, 51*t*
Antipsychotics, 52*t*
Antiretrovirals, 52*t*

Antirheumatics, 52*t*

Antituberculosis medications, 52*t*

Anxiety disorder, 33

Approved abbreviation list for diagnoses and terminology, 181–190

Arachidonic acid (AA), 97. *See also* Omega-3 fatty acids

ARBs (angiotensin II receptor blockers), 31

Aripiprazole, 34

Aspiration and enteral nutrition, 23

Aspirin, 32

Asthma, 42

BCAAs (branch chain amino acids), 37

Bed sores. *See* Pressure ulcers

Benadryl, 75

Beta blockers, 31

Binge eating disorder, 120–122

Biochemical data, 42, 43, 44–49*t*

Bioelectrical impedance analysis (BIA), 87

Bipolar disorder, 33

Birth defects, 99–100

Blood urea nitrogen (BUN), 44*t*

Body fat percentage, 86–88, 87–88*t*

Body mass index (BMI)
  adjusted body weight and, 13
  coronary artery bypass grafting and, 9
  as objective assessment tool, 85–86, 85*t*
  pediatric obesity, 123–126, 124–125*f*

Body parts missing, 8

Bone mineral density, 90–91

Braden Scale, 15

Branch chain amino acids (BCAAs), 37

Branched chain ketoaciduria, 118–119

Breastfeeding, 103–104, 110

Bronchitis, 42

Buddhism, dietary practices, 66

Bulimia nervosa, 120

BUN (blood urea nitrogen), 44*t*

CABG (coronary artery bypass grafting), 8–10

Caffeine, 21

Calcium, 44*t*

Calcium oxalate renal stones, 7

Caloric needs
  adolescents, 126, 126*t*
  children, 112, 113*t*, 126, 126*t*
  determination of, 132, 133*t*
  developmental disabilities and, 117
  infants, 112, 113*t*
  parenteral nutrition and, 25
  during pregnancy, 96

Calorie count study, 82–84, 84*t*

CAM (complementary and alternative medicine), 69–74

Cancer, 17

Carbohydrates, 25, 27, 35–36

Cardiac cachexia, 32

Cardiovascular review, 28–33
  angina, 29–30
  cerebral vascular accidents, 28–29
  congestive heart failure, 29
  hypertension, 30–31
  medications, 31
  myocardial infarction, 29–30
  obesity, 31

Care plan
  creation of, 134–142
  discharge instructions, 142
  follow-up plans, 139–140
  goals, 136
  interventions/recommendations, 136–137
  monitoring procedures, 137–138
  oral feeding transition, 138–139
  outcome evaluation, 139
  patient education, 140–142, 141*t*
  sample, 135*t*

Catabolism, 90

Catholicism, dietary practices, 68

Centers for Medicare and Medicaid Services (CMS), 15

Cerebral vascular accidents (CVAs), 28–29

Chart review, 3–57. *See also specific diagnoses and interventions*
  biochemical data, 43, 44–49*t*
  cardiovascular, 28–33
  food allergies and intolerance, 74–77, 76–77*f*

gastrointestinal review, 17–28
infectious diseases, 34–40
medical diagnosis, 4–5
medications, 31, 43–53, 50–53*t*
musculoskeletal review, 40–41
psychiatric review, 33–34
psychosocial review, 41
pulmonary, 41–42
skin integrity, 15–17
surgical review and history, 5–12
weight history, 12–15
CHD (coronary heart disease), 29–31
CHF (congestive heart failure), 29
Children. *See also* Pediatric assessment
calorie and protein requirements, 112,
113*t*, 126, 126*t*
eating disorders, 119–123
expected weight and height gains, 112,
112*t*, 114–115*f*
Chloride, 45*t*
Cholesterol, 30, 32, 36, 49*t*
Chromium, 73
Chronic kidney disease, 156–157*t*
Chronic liver infection, 35
Chronic malnutrition. *See* Malnutrition
Chronic obstructive pulmonary disease
(COPD), 42
Cirrhosis, 35
Clostridium difficile (c-diff), 19
Coenzyme Q10, 73
Cognition of patient, 145–146
Colostomy, 11–12, 163–164*t*
Complementary and alternative medicine
(CAM), 69–74
Congestive heart failure (CHF), 29, 155*t*
Constipation
anticonvulsants and, 40
antidepressants and, 33
developmental disabilities and, 116
enteral nutrition and, 22
gastrointestinal review, 20–21
during pregnancy, 101
Contraindications for enteral and parenteral
nutrition, 22, 25

COPD (chronic obstructive pulmonary
disease), 42
Coronary artery bypass grafting (CABG), 8–10
Coronary heart disease (CHD), 29–31
Coumadin (warfarin), 32, 71
C-reactive protein (CRP), 30
Creatinine, 44*t*
Culture and dietary practices, 64–66
CVAs (cerebral vascular accidents), 28–29
Cystic fibrosis, 63

Decubitis ulcers. *See* Pressure ulcers
Dehydration. *See also* Fluid requirements
delayed wound healing and, 17
eating disorders and, 122
enteral nutrition and, 23
parenteral nutrition and, 28
vomiting and, 19–20
Delayed wound healing, 15–17
Dementia, 34
Depression
during pregnancy, 93, 100
psychiatric review, 33
weight loss and, 10
Developmental disabilities, 116–117, 117*t*
DHA (docosahexaenoic acid), 97. *See also*
Omega-3 fatty acids
Diabetes
fasting and, 69
gestational, 102–103, 160*t*
heart disease and, 29
herbal supplements for, 72–73
pancreatectomy and, 10–11
patient education, 158–160*t*
race and ethnicity and, 63
Diagnosis
abbreviation list for, 181–190
chart review, 4–5
nutrition, 3
Diarrhea
colostomy and, 12
enteral nutrition and, 22
gastrointestinal review, 18–20
ileostomy and, 12

Dietary fiber, 21, 32, 96
Diet history interview, 60–61
Digoxin, 31
Dilantin (phenytoin), 24
Diphenhydramine, 75
Direct observation study, 81–82, 150
Discharge instructions, 142
Distal pancreatectomy, 10
Diuretics, 31, 51*t*
Diverticulosis, 162–163*t*
Docosahexaenoic acid (DHA), 97. *See also*
    Omega-3 fatty acids
Documentation
    guidelines, 174–176
    malpractice issues and, 172–174
    mechanics of, 176–178
    medical record as legal document, 172
    Nutrition Care Process model, 178–179
    purpose of, 171–172
Drug use, 93, 99, 104. *See also* Medications
"Dumping syndrome," 6
Dysphagia, 116

Eating disorders
    anorexia nervosa, 18, 119–120
    binge eating disorder, 120–122
    bulimia nervosa, 120
Eclampsia, 101–102
Education level of patient, 41, 146–147
Electrolytes, 25, 39
Emesis. *See* Nausea and vomiting
Emphysema, 42
End-stage liver disease (ESLD), 37,
    161–162*t*
Enteral nutrition
    chart review, 21–24
    complications, 22–24
    gastrointestinal review, 21–24
    for low-birthweight infants, 109, 111*t*
    patient education, 165*t*
    transition to oral feeding, 138–139
EpiPen Auto-Injector, 75
ESLD (end-stage liver disease), 37, 161–162*t*

Ethnicity
    body fat percentage and, 87–88*t*
    disease relationships and, 63–64

Failure to thrive assessment, 112–116, 116*t*
Fasting, 66–69
FDA (Food and Drug Administration), 72,
    98
Fecal impaction, 20–21
Ferritin, 46*t*
Fetal growth retardation, 99–100
Feverfew, 71
FFQ (food frequency questionnaire), 62–63
Fiber. *See* Dietary fiber
Fibrates, 51*t*
Fluid requirements
    determination of, 132–134
    enteral nutrition and, 23
    during pregnancy, 97
    short bowel syndrome and, 6–7
Follow-up plans, 139–140
Food allergies and intolerance, 74–77,
    76–77*f,* 100
Food Allergy and Anaphylaxis Network, 75
Food and Drug Administration (FDA), 72,
    98
Food frequency questionnaire (FFQ), 62–63
Food security, 147
Full-term infants, assessment, 110*t,*
    112, 112*t*

Gallstones, 6
Garlic, 71, 73
Gastric bypass surgery, 5–6, 164*t*
Gastric residual volume, 23–24
Gastroesophageal reflux disease (GERD), 101
Gastrointestinal review, 17–28
    constipation and fecal impaction, 20–21
    enteral nutrition, 21–24
    nausea and vomiting, 18
    parenteral nutrition, 24–28
    stools and diarrhea, 18–20
Gastroschisis, 99

Gaucher's disease, 64
GERD (gastroesophageal reflux disease), 101
Gestational diabetes, 102–103, 160*t*
Ginger, 71
Ginkgo biloba, 71
Ginseng, 71
Glucocorticoids and delayed wound
    healing, 17
Glucosamine, 72
Glucose, 48*t*, 88, 89*t*
Glycosylated hemoglobin, 48*t*
Gynoid obesity, 86

HAART (highly active antiretroviral
    therapy), 39
Hand-grip strength test, 37
HDL. *See* High-density lipoprotein
Heartburn, 101
Heart disease, 29–31
Height
    ideal body weight and, 13
    infants and children
        expected gains, 112, 112*t*, 114–115*f*
Hematocrit, 46*t*
Hemoglobin, 46*t*
Heparin, 71
Hepatitis A, 34
Hepatitis B, 35, 63
Hepatitis C, 35–37
Herbal supplement usage
    for diabetes, 72–73
    interview, 69–74, 70–71*t*
    medication interactions, 71–72
Hereditary hemochromatosis (HHC), 63
High-density lipoprotein (HDL), 30, 32, 48*t*
Highly active antiretroviral therapy
    (HAART), 39
Hinduism, dietary practices, 67
HIV/AIDS
    chart review, 37–38
    delayed wound healing and, 17
    heart disease and, 29
    patient education, 157–158*t*

Homelessness, 147
Homocystinuria, 117–118
H¹-Antagonists, 52*t*
Hydration. *See* Fluid requirements
Hyperbilirubinemia, 102
Hyperglycemia, 27, 28
Hyperlipidemia, 39, 154–155*t*
Hypertension, 30–31, 32, 101–102, 154*t*
Hypertonic dehydration, 28
Hypertriglyceridemia, 28
Hypnotics, 53*t*
Hypoalbuminemia, 9, 42
Hypocalcemia, 102
Hypoglycemia, 11

IBD (inflammatory bowel disease), 161*t*
Ideal body weight determination, 8, 13
Ileostomy, 11–12, 163–164*t*
Inborn errors of amino acid metabolism,
    117–119
Indirect calorimetry, 88–89
Infants. *See also* Pediatric assessment
    calorie and protein requirements, 112,
        113*t*
    expected weight and height gains, 112,
        112*t*, 114–115*f*
Infectious diseases
    chart review, 34–40
    hepatitis A, 34
    hepatitis B, 35
    hepatitis C, 35–37
    HIV/AIDS, 37–38
    pneumonia, 39–40
    pulmonary tuberculosis, 38–39
    urinary tract infection, 38
Inflammatory bowel disease (IBD), 161*t*
Informed consent, 175
International Normalized Ratio (INR), 32
International Osteoporosis Foundation, 91
Interventions. *See also specific interventions*
    in care plan, 136–137
    defined, 4
    pregnancy, 100–103

Interview, 59–80
  culture and dietary practices, 64–66
  diet history, 60–61
  as education evaluation, 150
  food frequency questionnaire, 62–63
  herbal supplement usage, 69–74, 70–71*t*
  race/ethnicity and disease relationships,
    63–64
  religion and dietary practices, 66–69
  24-hour recall, 62
  weight history, 61–62
Intravenous hyperalimentation (IVH), 24
Islam, dietary practices, 67
I-tal food, 68

Judaism, dietary practices, 67

Kava, 72
Kidney stones, 7

Lactation, 103–104
Lasix, 31, 32
Laxatives, 53*t*
LBW (low-birthweight) infants, 108–112,
    110–111*t*
LDL. *See* Low-density lipoprotein
Legal aspects of documentation, 171–180
Lipids, 25, 30
Liqiang 4 dietary supplement, 72
Literacy level of patient, 146–147
Lithium, 33, 51*t*
Liver disease, 34–37
Low-birthweight (LBW) infants, 108–112,
    110–111*t*
Low-density lipoprotein (LDL), 30, 32, 49*t*
Lupus, 63–64

Magnesium, 47*t*, 73
Malnutrition
  delayed wound healing and, 17
  eating disorders and, 122
  enteral nutrition for, 21
  hepatitis and, 36

  in infants and children, 113–114
  maternal, 99
  pulmonary function and, 41–42
  Waterlow criteria for, 113, 116*t*
  weight loss, 14, 15*t*
Malpractice and documentation issues,
    172–174
Manic depressive disorder, 33
Maple syrup urine disease (MSUD), 118–
    119
Mastectomy, 8
Maternal malnutrition, 99
MCTs (medium chain triglycerides), 11, 37
Mean corpuscular hemoglobin (MCH), 46*t*
Mean corpuscular hemoglobin concentration
    (MCHC), 47*t*
Mean corpuscular volume (MCV), 47*t*
Medical nutrition therapy (MNT), 103
Medications. *See also specific medications*
  anticonvulsant, 40
  cardiovascular review, 31
  chart review, 31, 43–53, 50–53*t*
  constipation caused by, 20
  delayed wound healing and, 17
  herbal supplement interactions, 71–72
  parenteral nutrition and, 25
  triglyceride increase caused by, 29
Medium chain triglycerides (MCTs), 11, 37
Mental retardation, 116–117
Mercury, 98
Minerals
  gastric bypass surgery and, 6
  parenteral nutrition and, 25
  pregnancy needs, 96–97
  pressure ulcers and, 17
  short bowel syndrome and, 7
Missing body parts, 8
MNT (medical nutrition therapy), 103
Monitoring procedures, 4, 137–138
Mormonism, dietary practices, 68
MSUD (maple syrup urine disease), 118–119
Muscle relaxants, 53*t*
Muscular dystrophy, 40

Musculoskeletal review, 40–41
Myocardial infarction, 29–30

Nasogastric tube (NGT), 21
National Cancer Institute, 10
National Center for Complementary and
    Alternative Medicine, 72
National Health and Nutritional
    Examination Survey (NHANES), 62
National Institute for Clinical Excellence
    (NICE), 27
Nausea and vomiting, 6, 18, 100–101
Neonatal hypoglycemia, 102
NGT (nasogastric tube), 21
Niacin, 32, 51t
Nitrogen balance, 89–90
Noncompliance, 174–175
Nonsteroidal anti-inflammatory drugs
    (NSAIDs), 53t
Nutrient requirements, 96–98, 132–134,
    133t. *See also* Caloric needs; Protein
    needs
Nutrition assessment, 3
Nutrition Care Process
    as documentation model, 178–179
    intervention, 131
    interview, 59
    monitoring, 137–138
    objective assessment tools, 81
    outcome evaluation, 139
    steps for, 3–4
Nutrition diagnosis. *See* Diagnosis
Nutrition evaluation, 4, 139
Nutrition intervention, defined, 4. *See also*
    Interventions
Nutrition monitoring, 4, 137–138

Obesity
    android vs. gynoid, 86
    cardiovascular review, 31
    coronary heart disease and, 31
    developmental disabilities and, 116
    pediatric assessment, 123–126, 124–125f

Objective assessment tools, 81–92
    body fat percentage, 86–88, 87–88t
    body mass index, 85–86, 85t
    bone mineral density, 90–91
    calorie count study, 82–84, 84t
    direct observation study, 81–82
    indirect calorimetry, 88–89
    nitrogen balance, 89–90
    waist circumference and waist-to-hip
        ratio, 86
OGT (orogastric tube), 21
Omega-3 fatty acids, 71, 73, 97–98
Oral feeding, 109–112, 138–139. *See also*
    Enteral nutrition; Parenteral nutrition
Oral hypoglycemics, 53t
Oral rehydration solutions (ORSs), 7
Orogastric tube (OGT), 21
Osteoporosis, 90–91, 116
Outcome evaluation, 4, 139
Overhydration, 23, 133–134

Pancreatectomy, 10–11
Parenteral nutrition
    chart review, 24–28, 26f
    components of, 25
    contraindications, 25
    formula calculations, 25–27
    for low-birthweight infants, 109, 111t
    patient education, 166t
    qualifications for, 24
Patient education, 145–152
    in care plan, 140–142, 141t
    chronic kidney disease, 156–157t
    colostomy, 163–164t
    congestive heart failure, 155t
    diabetes, 158–160t
    diverticulosis, 162–163t
    end-stage liver disease, 161–162t
    evaluation of, 149–152
    gastric bypass surgery, 164t
    gestational diabetes, 160t
    HIV/AIDS, 157–158t
    home enteral nutrition, 165t

home parenteral nutrition, 166*t*
hyperlipidemia, 154–155*t*
hypertension, 154*t*
ileostomy, 163–164*t*
inflammatory bowel disease, 161*t*
learning objectives, 149
short bowel syndrome, 162*t*
specific conditions, 154–166*t*
PCBs (polychlorinated biphenyls), 98
PCM (protein-calorie malnutrition), 36
Pediatric assessment, 107–128
developmental disability, 116–117, 117*t*
eating disorders, 119–123
failure to thrive, 112–116, 116*t*
full-term infants, 110*t*, 112, 112*t*
homocystinuria, 117–118
inborn errors of amino acid metabolism,
117–119
low-birthweight infants, 108–112,
110–111*t*
maple syrup urine disease, 118–119
mental retardation, 116–117
obesity, 123–126, 124–125*f*
phenylketonuria, 118
terminology, 107
Percutaneous endoscopic gastrostomy (PEG),
21. *See also* Enteral nutrition
Percutaneous endoscopic jejunostomy (PEJ),
21. *See also* Enteral nutrition
Peripheral parenteral nutrition (PPN), 24
Phenylketonuria (PKU), 118
Phenytoin, 24
Phosphorus, 45*t*
Pneumonia, 39–40
Polychlorinated biphenyls (PCBs), 98
Potassium, 45*t*
PPN (peripheral parenteral nutrition), 24
Prealbumin, 44*t*
Preeclampsia, 101–102
Preexisting medical conditions, 100
Pregnancy, 93–106
caloric needs, 96
complications and interventions, 100–103

constipation, 101
dietary assessment, 93–95, 94–95*f*
dietary fiber, 96
eclampsia, 101–102
fluid requirements, 97
gastroesophageal reflux disease, 101
gestational diabetes, 102–103
heartburn, 101
lactation, 103–104
nausea and vomiting, 100–101
nutritional needs, 96–98
omega-3 fatty acids, 97–98
preeclampsia, 101–102
protein needs, 96
risk factors, 99–100
vitamins and minerals, 96–97
weight gain, 98, 98*t*
Pressure ulcers, 15, 16*t*, 17, 29
Pre-term infants, 108–112, 110–111*t*
Probiotics, 19–20
Protein-calorie malnutrition (PCM), 36
Protein needs
adolescents, 126, 126*t*
children, 112, 113*t*, 126, 126*t*
determination of, 132, 133*t*
infants, 112, 113*t*
parenteral nutrition and, 25, 28
during pregnancy, 96
Proton pump inhibitors, 51*t*
Psychiatric review, 33–34
Psychosocial review, 41
Pulmonary chart review, 41–42
Pulmonary tuberculosis (TB), 38–39
Pyridoxine, 118

Quality indicators, 134

Race
body fat percentage and, 87–88*t*
disease relationships and, 63–64
Rastafarianism, dietary practices, 68
Recommendations in care plan, 136–137
Red blood cells (RBC), 46*t*

Red yeast rice products, 72
Refeeding syndrome, 22–23, 27
Religion and dietary practices, 66–69
Renal function, 32
Respiratory quotient (RQ), 42, 88, 89*t*
Rifampin, 39
Risk factors
    chronic obstructive pulmonary disease, 42
    coronary heart disease, 29
    delayed wound healing, 15–17
    gestational diabetes, 102
    osteoporosis, 90–91
    pregnancy, 99–100
Roman Catholicism, dietary practices, 68
RQ. *See* Respiratory quotient

St. John's wort, 71
Sedatives, 53*t*
Selective serotonin reuptake inhibitors
    (SSRIs), 100
Seventh-Day Adventists, dietary practices, 68
SGA (subjective global assessment), 37
Short bowel syndrome, 6–7, 162*t*
Sickle cell anemia, 64
Skin fold thickness, 87
Skin integrity, 15–17
SLE (systemic lupus erythematosus), 63–64
Smoking
    body mass index and, 86
    chronic obstructive pulmonary disease
      and, 42
    heart disease and, 29
    hypertension and, 30
    pregnancy and, 99
Socioeconomic factors, 41
Sodium, 44*t*
SSRIs (selective serotonin reuptake
    inhibitors), 100
Stages of Change Model, 148
Statins, 51*t*
Steatorrhea, 7, 11, 37
Steroids, 53*t*
Stools, 12, 18–20

Strokes, 28–29
Subjective global assessment (SGA), 37
Surgical review and history, 5–12
    colostomy, 11–12
    coronary artery bypass grafting, 8–10
    gastric bypass, 5–6
    ileostomy, 11–12
    missing body parts, 8
    pancreatectomy, 10–11
    short bowel syndrome, 6–7
Systemic lupus erythematosus (SLE), 63–64

Tay-Sachs disease, 64
TB (pulmonary tuberculosis), 38–39
Terminology
    abbreviation list for, 181–190
    pediatric assessment, 107
Thalassemia, 64
Thyroid medications, 53*t*
Total iron binding capacity, 47*t*
Total parenteral nutrition (TPN), 7, 24, 109.
    See also Parenteral nutrition
Transferrin Test, 47*t*
Transtheoretical Model, 148
Triglycerides, 36, 49*t*
Tuberculosis, 38–39
24-hour recall interview, 62

Urea urinary nitrogen (UUN), 90
Urinary tract infection, 38
Usual body weight (UBW), 14

Very-low-birthweight (VLBW) infants, 109
Vitamins
    gastric bypass surgery and, 6
    parenteral nutrition and, 25
    pregnancy needs, 96–97
    pressure ulcers and, 17
    short bowel syndrome and, 7
    vegetarian diets and, 69

Waist circumference and waist-to-hip ratio,
    31, 86

Warfarin, 32, 71

Waterlow criteria for malnutrition, 113, 116*t*

Weight

    adjusted body weight determination, 13–14

    chart review, 12–15

    ideal body weight determination, 13

    infants and children, expected gains, 112, 112*t*, 114–115*f*

    interview for history, 61–62

    pregnancy gains, 98, 98*t*

    pressure ulcers, 15, 16*t*, 17

    weight change determination, 14–15, 15*t*

Whipple procedure, 10